D0182913

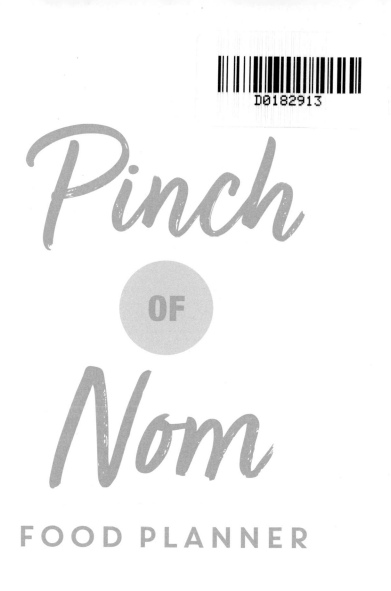

Pinch OF Nom

FOOD PLANNER

First published 2019 by Bluebird
an imprint of Pan Macmillan
20 New Wharf Road, London N1 9RR
Associated companies throughout the world
www.panmacmillan.com

ISBN   978-1-5290-2306-0

Copyright © Kate Allinson, Kay Featherstone, Laura Davis 2019

The right of Kate Allinson, Kay Featherstone and Laura Davis to be identified as the authors of this work has been asserted by them in accordance with the Copyright, Designs and Patents Act 1988.

All rights reserved. No part of this publication may be reproduced, stored in a retrieval system, or transmitted, in any form, or by any means (electronic, mechanical, photocopying, recording or otherwise) without the prior written permission of the publisher.

Pan Macmillan does not have any control over, or any responsibility for, any author or third-party websites referred to in or on this book.

1 3 5 7 9 8 6 4 2

A CIP catalogue record for this book is available from the British Library.

Printed and bound in Italy.

Publisher Carole Tonkinson
Managing Editor Martha Burley
Senior Production Controller Sarah Badhan
Art Direction, Design and Illustration Emma Wells, Nic&Lou Design
Additional illustrations Shutterstock

This book is sold subject to the condition that it shall not, by way of trade or otherwise, be lent, hired out, or otherwise circulated without the publisher's prior consent in any form of binding or cover other than that in which it is published and without a similar condition including this condition being imposed on the subsequent purchaser.

Visit www.panmacmillan.com to read more about all our books and to buy them. You will also find features, author interviews and news of any author events, and you can sign up for e-newsletters so that you're always first to hear about our new releases.

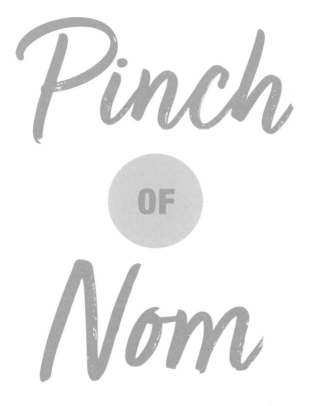

Pinch OF Nom

FOOD PLANNER

Includes 26 Recipes

bluebird
books for life

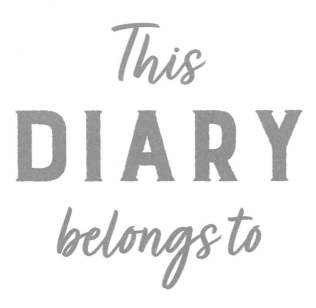

This

DIARY

belongs to

....

....

CONTENTS

This book is yours, so use this page to scribble down page numbers in this book – so you can easily refer to a particular week or day of progress, or recipe you love.

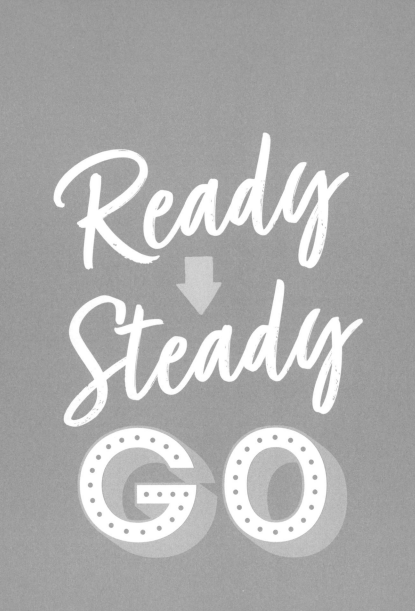

WELCOME TO THE
Pinch OF Nom
FOOD PLANNER

The best way to keep track of success on any healthy-eating plan is to record everything you're eating. Using this handy all-in-one planner, you can refer to your complete food intake on a daily basis, while also being able to look back on previous days and weeks to highlight your best meal choices. We've tried to make this planner as accessible as possible, meaning you can use it whether you're simply calorie counting or following one of the UK's most popular diet plans. This planner is the perfect tool for keeping track, regardless of the diet plan you are following.

Pinch of Nom started out as a small idea, by Kate and Kay, to share their slimming recipes with a small number of friends and family. While the recipes are still at the heart of everything Pinch of Nom does, the community that has grown has been an amazing and unexpected bonus! Now with a huge online following of over 1.4 million Facebook Page likes and a Facebook Group of around 800,000 people, the Pinch of Nom community offers support and tips, spurring on each others' weight-loss journeys. Kate and Kay only ever wanted to help others with their recipes and the Pinch of Nom platform.

How to
USE THE PLANNER

We've been listening to the Pinch of Nom community and this is the result: a useful and functional food planner. With added recipes to boot! It is a beautiful, portable journal for jotting down all of the helpful things for any weight-loss journey.

Start this planner by writing down your main aims, plans and goals for the next 26 weeks (or 6 months!). This is *your* planner – it needs to work for you and inspire you as much as it helps keep track of your food intake. While that may seem like a big ask, just recording your initial hopes for the next 6 months will give you something to reflect on and reminds you where you want to be. Seeing your aspirations in your own writing will have a great impact on your motivation to succeed.

We've given you options to enter your weight at the start of each week, as well as space to jot down your thoughts, goals or aims, plus anything you did well the previous week or you want to improve on. We strongly advise you take a little time out each week to complete these sections. Not only is it a good way to focus on planning for your upcoming week, but it also gives you a chance to reflect on both the negatives and, more importantly, the positives from the week gone by. This will stand you in good stead going forwards so you're not repeating mistakes, but you're also continuing to do things that have had a positive impact on your weight loss. Although it sounds like a simple step, this mindful approach to your weeks will make a big difference if you use the sections as suggested.

From first-hand experience, we know how hard it is to stay motivated with your eyes on that target. We've tried to incorporate that same sense of community and support that has developed online by providing motivational thoughts and phrases that will hopefully keep you inspired and focused on reaching your goal.

'I've been using the planner every day! It's fab! It's really clear and easy to fill in. I love that there's plenty of space to be able to write down what you have eaten.' CHERYL

The **15**
TREATS RULE

Let's not get carried away here; we're not suggesting you can eat 15 chocolate gateaux a day … sadly! The treats aren't necessarily supposed to be seen as individual treats. They're more a breakdown to give easy ways of counting any calories that belong to processed foods – i.e. not your fruits, vegetables, lean meats, fish and fresh, nutritious ingredients, which we believe you should be able to enjoy without counting the calories and without limiting yourself. Each treat should be seen as around 20 calories. So each day you could, for example, have 15 treats at 20 calories each. Or, on the other hand, each day you could have one treat at 300 calories. Or somewhere in-between with a mix of treats. If 300 calories of treats a day sounds like a lot, you have to remember that any food that isn't fruit, vegetables, lean meats, fish and other fresh ingredients (herbs, eggs etc), must be counted in your treats section. So use those treats wisely – they're there to balance out your diet with fats and carbohydrates you need, but they require some thought. Make sure you're recording them fully – a few missed treats can add up over a week!

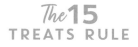

Drinking
WATER

In the UK, NHS experts advise that we should be drinking around 1.2 litres of water, which equates to around 8 glasses per day. So we've given you 8 water drops to fill up each time you have a glass of water. This simple marking tool is a great way to keep on plan with your water consumption, which studies say can directly help with weight loss. Firstly, often thirst can be mistaken for hunger, and secondly, studies have found that the body's metabolism works at a higher rate when fully hydrated. All great reasons to make a note of how much you're drinking a day. Not to mention being able to congratulate yourself when all 8 drops are filled!

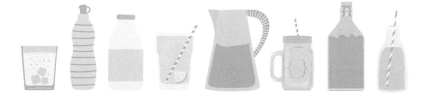

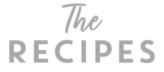

The RECIPES

We've included brand-new, weekly recipes, created just for you. These recipes are exclusive to this planner – they can't be found anywhere else! Compatible with the UK's major diet plans, the recipes are also calorie-friendly without compromising on taste.

At the heart of everything we do, the recipes are by far the most important and precious to us. Each recipe in this planner has been created to give you ideas that can be used again and again throughout the month.

To give you more pages for writing up your goals and food plans, the book does not have any photographs of the recipes, however you can find them on the Pinch of Nom website (www.pinchofnom.com/planner).

The recipes have been tested by our wonderful group of taste testers who were hand-picked from our very own Facebook Group. We wanted to be completely sure that each recipe works and tastes just as good to you as it did when we created it! We also wanted to be sure that the recipes work in unison with people following particular weight-loss plans, as well as calorie counting. We're really proud of the recipes in this planner and we hope you find them useful as part of your cooking and meal planning routine.

Each of the recipes falls into a category that is explained opposite. We hope this helps with your meal planning for each week and we also hope you enjoy making them as much as we enjoyed developing them!

'I love the recipes! So unique in comparison to other planners. Big thumbs up from me.' TERESA

Everyday Light

At Pinch of Nom, we believe in the ethos of 'everything in moderation'. With this in mind, our Everyday Light recipes are those you can have at any time: they're easy on the calories, filling and perfect for every day. You may notice some of these recipes are higher in calories than those in the other categories. The reason for this is that some calories are 'used up' on vegetables and other ingredients that conform to zero point-style foods applicable to the UK's most popular diet programmes.

Weekly Indulgence

These are recipes you can add to your weekly meal plans but have one or two ingredients that make them slightly more indulgent, so should be used in moderation. A good basis of any diet should be that you don't have to miss out on enjoying dinner parties or the odd treat here or there.

Special Occasion

Our Special Occasion recipes have your back! Lower in calories than regular desserts, snacks or treats, this section still comes out tops against high-calorie versions. However, the aforementioned ethos of 'everything in moderation' should come to mind with these. Save these recipes for pushing the boat out and for … you guessed it … special occasions!

Calories and Values

Our calorie counts are all worked out per individual serving. This does not include accompaniments for specific recipes, such as rice or potatoes. This is because we give these notes as a serving suggestion only. You can easily swap out rice and pasta for veggie low-calorie alternatives, such as cauliflower rice.

We have not included 'values' from mainstream diet programmes as these are ever-changing and we want this book to be a resource that is always up to date.

Our Recipe Icons

Each recipe also displays a set of easily-identifiable icons; explained below.

V Suitable for vegetarians

F Suitable for freezing. (For all freezer-friendly recipes, we recommend defrosting completely before heating until piping hot.)

GF Suitable for those following a gluten-free diet

Week One

CHANGE +/-

CURRENT WEIGHT

THIS WEEK I WOULD LIKE TO ACHIEVE

LAST WEEK, THESE THINGS WENT WELL...

REMINDERS FOR THIS WEEK

◯ **PLANNED MEALS**

◯ **SHOPPING DONE**

◯ **PLANNED EXERCISE**

Day One

BREAKFAST

LUNCH

DINNER

SNACK 1

SNACK 2

TREATS

WATER

Day Two

BREAKFAST

LUNCH

DINNER

SNACK 1

SNACK 2

TREATS

WATER

WEEK 1

Day Three

BREAKFAST

LUNCH

DINNER

SNACK 1

SNACK 2

TREATS

WATER

Day Four

BREAKFAST

LUNCH

DINNER

SNACK 1

SNACK 2

TREATS

WATER

Day Five

BREAKFAST

LUNCH

DINNER

SNACK 1

SNACK 2

TREATS

WATER

Day Six

BREAKFAST

LUNCH

DINNER

SNACK 1

SNACK 2

TREATS

WATER

Day Seven

BREAKFAST

LUNCH

DINNER

SNACK 1

SNACK 2

TREATS

WATER

VEGGIE LASAGNE

🕐 **10 MINS** | 🍲 **1 HOUR** | 🔥 **451 KCAL** PER SERVING

When we introduced this recipe to our taste testers, we had multiple comments saying it was the best slimming lasagne recipe they had tried. We're so proud of this hearty, delicious and utterly decadent-tasting recipe, packed full of vegetables and bulked out with 'meaty' lentils. We think you will agree with our taste testers!

Special Occasion

V **F**

SERVES 6

low-calorie cooking spray
2 large white onions,
    finely chopped
1 celery stick, finely chopped
1 carrot, finely chopped
4 garlic cloves, finely chopped
2 courgettes, finely chopped
1 red pepper, halved,
    deseeded and diced
6 white mushrooms,
    thinly sliced
2 x 400g tins green
    lentils, drained
1 tbsp dried oregano
1 tbsp dried basil
4 tbsp balsamic vinegar
1 red wine stock pot
1 tsp Marmite
1 x 400g tin chopped tomatoes
4 tbsp tomato puree
200ml vegetable stock
    (1 vegetable stock
    cube dissolved in
    200ml boiling water)

Spray a large frying pan that has a lid with low-calorie cooking spray and place over a medium heat. Add the onions, celery, carrot and garlic to the pan and cook for a few minutes until they start to soften and the onions start to turn translucent. Add the courgettes and pepper, stir, then add the mushrooms and spray with some more low-calorie cooking spray. Fry for about 5 minutes, mixing occasionally.

Add the lentils, oregano, basil, balsamic vinegar, wine stock pot, Marmite, tinned tomatoes, 2 tablespoons of the tomato puree and the vegetable stock to the pan and stir well. Cover and simmer for 20–30 minutes until thickened slightly and a bit deeper in colour. Meanwhile, preheat the oven to 200°C (fan 180°/gas mark 6).

Stir the spinach and the remaining tomato puree through the sauce and season to taste with salt and pepper.

Spread a layer of the mixture on the bottom of a very large ovenproof dish, then add a layer of lasagne sheets. Repeat until you reach the top of the dish, ending with a layer of lasagne sheets. Make sure you leave enough room for the white sauce.

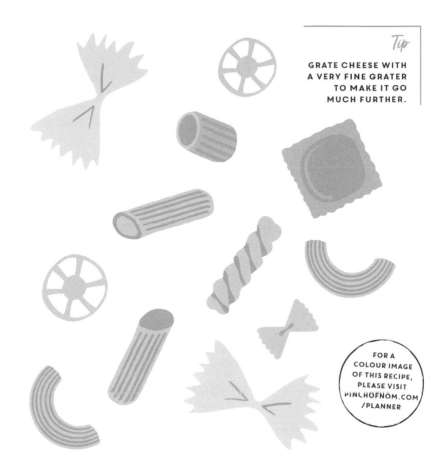

Tip

GRATE CHEESE WITH
A VERY FINE GRATER
TO MAKE IT GO
MUCH FURTHER.

FOR A
COLOUR IMAGE
OF THIS RECIPE,
PLEASE VISIT
PINCHOFNOM.COM
/PLANNER

handful of spinach leaves,
   hard stalks discarded and
   roughly chopped
sea salt and freshly ground
   black pepper
10 dried lasagne sheets

FOR THE WHITE SAUCE
500g fat-free natural yoghurt
2 medium eggs
½ tsp English mustard powder
1 tsp onion granules
120g reduced-fat
   Cheddar, grated

To make the white sauce, mix the yoghurt, eggs, mustard powder and onion granules in a bowl and season with salt and pepper. Beat well to make sure the mixture is smooth. Pour this sauce over the top of the lasagne sheets, then sprinkle the grated cheese on top. Make sure the lasagne is shy from the top of the dish to avoid it spilling over in the oven.

Cook in the oven for 30 minutes, until bubbling and browning on top.

Remove from the oven and serve, or allow to cool and freeze in an airtight container.

21

Week Two

CHANGE +/-

CURRENT WEIGHT

THIS WEEK I WOULD LIKE TO ACHIEVE

LAST WEEK, THESE THINGS WENT WELL...

REMINDERS FOR THIS WEEK

○ PLANNED
MEALS

○ SHOPPING
DONE

○ PLANNED
EXERCISE

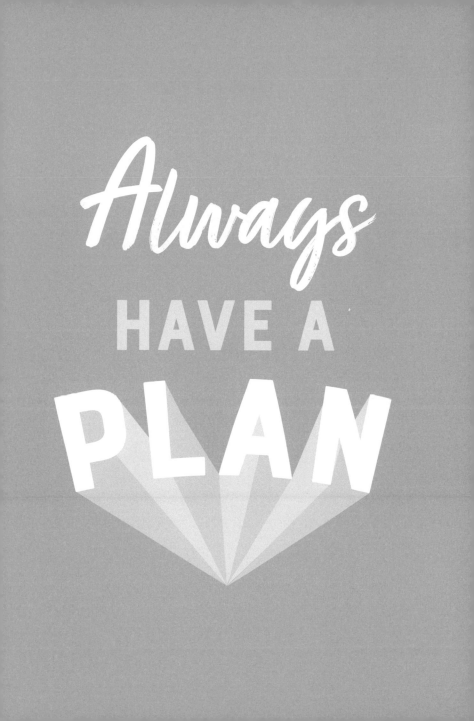

Day One

BREAKFAST

LUNCH

DINNER

SNACK 1

SNACK 2

TREATS

WATER

Day Two

BREAKFAST

LUNCH

DINNER

SNACK 1

SNACK 2

TREATS

WATER

Day Three

BREAKFAST

LUNCH

DINNER

SNACK 1

SNACK 2

TREATS

WATER

Day Four

BREAKFAST

LUNCH

DINNER

SNACK 1

SNACK 2

TREATS

WATER

Day Five

BREAKFAST

LUNCH

DINNER

SNACK 1

SNACK 2

TREATS

WATER

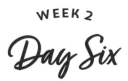

WEEK 2

Day Six

BREAKFAST

LUNCH

DINNER

SNACK 1

SNACK 2

TREATS

WATER

Day Seven

BREAKFAST

LUNCH

DINNER

SNACK 1

SNACK 2

TREATS

WATER

PIGS *in* POTATOES

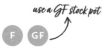

FOR A COLOUR IMAGE OF THIS RECIPE, PLEASE VISIT PINCHOFNOM.COM /PLANNER

🕐 **20 MINS** | 🍲 **40 MINS** | 🔥 **245 KCAL** PER SERVING

Pigs in potatoes taste as amazing as they sound! You'll find it hard to believe these salty, garlicky treats are low in calories. Use large, robust new potatoes to make the prep even easier.

Everyday Light

use a GF stock pot

F **GF**

SERVES 4

16 large new potatoes
1 medium egg
250g 5%-fat minced pork
1 tsp garlic granules
1 tsp onion granules
1 tsp English mustard powder
1 pork or chicken stock pot
sea salt and freshly ground
   black pepper
8 bacon medallions, cut into
   thin strips
low-calorie cooking spray
fresh chives, snipped, to
   garnish (optional)

Preheat the oven to 220°C (fan 200°/gas mark 7).

Cook the new potatoes in a saucepan of boiling water for about 20 minutes, or until they are tender. Drain and leave to cool.

Meanwhile, mix the egg, minced pork, garlic and onion granules, mustard and stock pot in a bowl and season with salt and pepper.

Cut the cooled potatoes in half and scoop out some of the middle, as if you are preparing stuffed potato skins.

Roughly chop or mash the potato flesh and mix it into the pork mixture, then spoon the pork mix into the potato skins. Drape the bacon strips over the tops of the potato skins.

Spray a baking tray with low-calorie cooking spray and place the potato skins on the tray, then spray the tops of the potatoes with more low-calorie cooking spray. Place the potatoes in the middle of the oven and cook for 20 minutes.

Remove from the oven and serve with chives sprinkled on top, if you like.

Tip

THESE MAKE A GREAT SIDE DISH OR PARTY APPETIZERS.

Week Three

CHANGE +/-

CURRENT WEIGHT

THIS WEEK I WOULD LIKE TO ACHIEVE

LAST WEEK, THESE THINGS WENT WELL...

REMINDERS FOR THIS WEEK

○ PLANNED MEALS

○ SHOPPING DONE

○ PLANNED EXERCISE

Day One

BREAKFAST

LUNCH

DINNER

SNACK 1

SNACK 2

TREATS

◐ ◐ ◐ ◐ ◐ ◐ ◐ ◐
◐ ◐ ◐ ◐ ◐ ◐ ◐

WATER

◇ ◇ ◇ ◇
◇ ◇ ◇ ◇

Day Two

BREAKFAST

LUNCH

DINNER

SNACK 1

SNACK 2

TREATS

WATER

Day Three

BREAKFAST

LUNCH

DINNER

SNACK 1

SNACK 2

TREATS

WATER

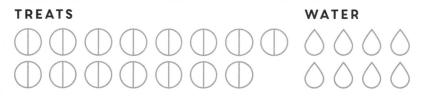

Day Four

BREAKFAST

LUNCH

DINNER

SNACK 1

SNACK 2

TREATS

WATER

Day Five

BREAKFAST

LUNCH

DINNER

SNACK 1

SNACK 2

TREATS

WATER

Day Six

BREAKFAST

LUNCH

DINNER

SNACK 1

SNACK 2

TREATS

WATER

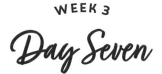

Day Seven

BREAKFAST

LUNCH

DINNER

SNACK 1

SNACK 2

TREATS

WATER

PAVLOVA

⏱ **15–20 MINS** | 🍲 **1 HOUR** PLUS COOLING | 🔥 **65 KCAL**

It's hard to believe you can indulge in a pavlova while following a slimming diet. However, a few substitutes turn this classic dessert into an indulgence that's lighter on calories than you might think. This is an occasional treat rather than an everyday pudding – once you try it you'll be counting down the days until your next dinner party!

 Special Occasion

GF

5 large egg whites,
    at room temperature
1 tsp cream of tartar
70g caster sugar
250g fat-free natural yoghurt
1 tbsp granulated sweetener
1 tsp vanilla extract
frozen (defrosted) or fresh
    berries of choice

Preheat the oven to 120°C (fan 100°/gas mark 1) and line a large baking sheet with baking parchment.

Place the egg whites in a very clean, dry mixing bowl, ensuring no egg yolk gets in the bowl with the whites. Whisk with an electric hand whisk until the egg whites form soft peaks, then add the cream of tartar and whisk to combine. Add the caster sugar, 1 tablespoon at a time, until fully combined. Continue whisking until the egg whites are stiff and glossy. When you feel the mixture, there should not be any grittiness from the sugar as it should all be dissolved. If it hasn't, whisk it for a little longer.

Carefully spoon the mixture onto the lined baking sheet and form it into a rough circle around 27cm (10in) in diameter. Create a slightly raised edge (2–3cm/¾–1¼in wide) to leave an area which your filling will sit in. Place in the oven and bake for 1 hour.

When the meringue is baked, turn off the oven, leaving the meringue on the baking sheet in the oven until completely cool. The meringue will keep for a few days in an airtight container at this point, if you want to make it in advance.

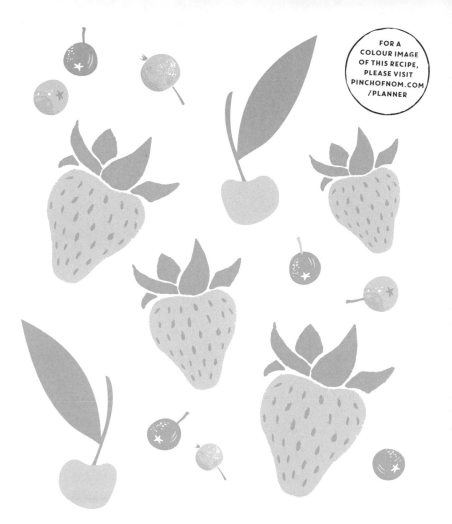

FOR A COLOUR IMAGE OF THIS RECIPE, PLEASE VISIT PINCHOFNOM.COM /PLANNER

To make the topping, mix together the yoghurt, sweetener and vanilla extract in a bowl and leave in the fridge until ready to assemble.

Prepare your fresh berries – strawberries, blueberries and raspberries work well.

When the meringue is completely cool, top it with the yoghurt mixture then top the yoghurt with fresh or defrosted berries. Serve immediately.

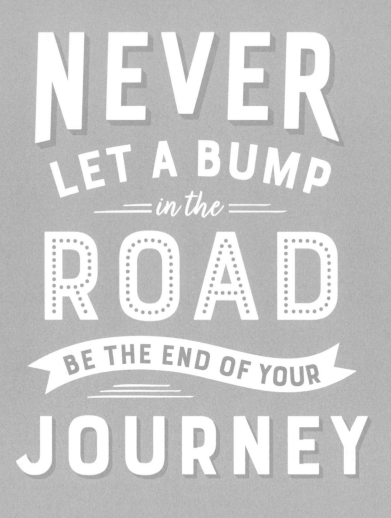

Week Four

CHANGE +/-

CURRENT WEIGHT

THIS WEEK I WOULD LIKE TO ACHIEVE

LAST WEEK, THESE THINGS WENT WELL...

REMINDERS FOR THIS WEEK

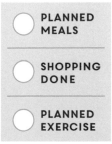

PLANNED
MEALS

SHOPPING
DONE

PLANNED
EXERCISE

Day One

BREAKFAST

LUNCH

DINNER

SNACK 1

SNACK 2

TREATS

WATER

Day Two

BREAKFAST

LUNCH

DINNER

SNACK 1

SNACK 2

TREATS

WATER

Day Three

BREAKFAST

LUNCH

DINNER

SNACK 1

SNACK 2

TREATS

WATER

Day Four

BREAKFAST

LUNCH

DINNER

SNACK 1

SNACK 2

TREATS

WATER

Day Five

BREAKFAST

LUNCH

DINNER

SNACK 1

SNACK 2

TREATS

⊖ ⊖ ⊖ ⊖ ⊖ ⊖ ⊖ ⊖

⊖ ⊖ ⊖ ⊖ ⊖ ⊖ ⊖

WATER

◇ ◇ ◇ ◇

◇ ◇ ◇ ◇

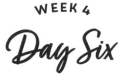

WEEK 4

Day Six

BREAKFAST

LUNCH

DINNER

SNACK 1

SNACK 2

TREATS

WATER

Day Seven

BREAKFAST

LUNCH

DINNER

SNACK 1

SNACK 2

TREATS

WATER

PORK *and* BACON PÂTÉ

🕐 **15 MINS** | 🍲 **10 MINS** | 💧 **299 KCAL** PER SERVING

Pâté isn't usually seen on a slimming-friendly recipe list, but this lean pork and bacon version uses generous seasoning to bring the very best pâté flavours to life. There's really no need for fatty, processed pâté when you have this recipe on hand!

Weekly Indulgence

SERVES 4

low-calorie cooking spray
1 onion, diced
2 garlic cloves, chopped
150g pig's liver (tough sinew removed), diced
200g lean pork (all visible fat removed), diced
100g bacon medallions, diced
½ tsp dried sage
pinch of cayenne pepper
sea salt and freshly ground black pepper
2 tbsp red wine vinegar
small handful of fresh parsley, chopped
1 tbsp fat-free Greek-style yoghurt

FOR A COLOUR IMAGE OF THIS RECIPE, PLEASE VISIT PINCHOFNOM.COM /PLANNER

Spray a frying pan with some low-calorie cooking spray, place over a medium heat then add the onion and garlic and cook for 4–5 minutes, or until they are soft and lightly browned.

Spray some more low-calorie cooking spray in the pan, then add the liver, pork and bacon. Stir in the sage and the cayenne and season with a little salt and pepper. Sauté until all the meat is cooked through. Add 1 tablespoon of the red wine vinegar and allow it to evaporate, then stir in the chopped parsley.

Transfer the mixture to a food processor or blender and blitz until you have a smooth pâté. Tip the pâté into a large bowl, then add the remaining vinegar and the yoghurt, and stir well.

Taste and check the seasoning, adding more salt and pepper if required. Place in an airtight container and refrigerate until you're ready to serve.

It will keep for a few days in the fridge, or you can freeze it in smaller portions and defrost as required.

Week Five

CHANGE +/-

CURRENT WEIGHT

THIS WEEK I WOULD LIKE TO ACHIEVE

LAST WEEK, THESE THINGS WENT WELL...

REMINDERS FOR THIS WEEK

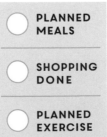

PLANNED MEALS

SHOPPING DONE

PLANNED EXERCISE

Day One

BREAKFAST

LUNCH

DINNER

SNACK 1

SNACK 2

TREATS

WATER

Day Two

BREAKFAST

LUNCH

DINNER

SNACK 1

SNACK 2

TREATS

WATER

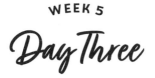

WEEK 5

Day Three

BREAKFAST

LUNCH

DINNER

SNACK 1

SNACK 2

TREATS

○ ○ ○ ○ ○ ○ ○ ○
○ ○ ○ ○ ○ ○

WATER

◇ ◇ ◇ ◇
◇ ◇ ◇ ◇

Day Four

BREAKFAST

LUNCH

DINNER

SNACK 1

SNACK 2

TREATS

WATER

Day Five

BREAKFAST

LUNCH

DINNER

SNACK 1

SNACK 2

TREATS

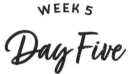

WATER

Day Six

BREAKFAST

LUNCH

DINNER

SNACK 1

SNACK 2

TREATS

WATER

Day Seven

BREAKFAST

LUNCH

DINNER

SNACK 1

SNACK 2

TREATS

WATER

Week Six

CHANGE +/-

CURRENT WEIGHT

THIS WEEK I WOULD LIKE TO ACHIEVE

LAST WEEK, THESE THINGS WENT WELL...

REMINDERS FOR THIS WEEK

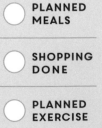

○ **PLANNED MEALS**

○ **SHOPPING DONE**

○ **PLANNED EXERCISE**

Day One

BREAKFAST

LUNCH

DINNER

SNACK 1

SNACK 2

TREATS

WATER

Day Two

BREAKFAST

LUNCH

DINNER

SNACK 1

SNACK 2

TREATS

WATER

Day Three

BREAKFAST

LUNCH

DINNER

SNACK 1

SNACK 2

TREATS

○ ○ ○ ○ ○ ○ ○ ○

○ ○ ○ ○ ○ ○ ○

WATER

◇ ◇ ◇ ◇

◇ ◇ ◇ ◇

Day Four

BREAKFAST

LUNCH

DINNER

SNACK 1

SNACK 2

TREATS

WATER

Day Five

BREAKFAST

LUNCH

DINNER

SNACK 1

SNACK 2

TREATS

WATER

Day Six

BREAKFAST

LUNCH

DINNER

SNACK 1

SNACK 2

TREATS

WATER

Day Seven

BREAKFAST

LUNCH

DINNER

SNACK 1

SNACK 2

TREATS

⊖ ⊖ ⊖ ⊖ ⊖ ⊖ ⊖ ⊖
⊖ ⊖ ⊖ ⊖ ⊖ ⊖ ⊖

WATER

◊ ◊ ◊ ◊
◊ ◊ ◊ ◊

BEEF *and* MUSHROOM CASSEROLE

🕐 **15 MINS** | 🍲 **VARIABLE** SEE BELOW | 🔥 **367 KCAL** PER SERVING

There's nothing more warming and hearty than a good casserole. The classic British combination of beef and mushroom gives huge depth of flavour to this traditional dish. The potato ingeniously thickens the dish and makes it more filling, and both slicing and dicing it gives the casserole added texture.

Everyday Light

---

use GF stock cubes

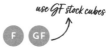

SERVES 4

2 beef stock cubes (plus 1 beef stock pot for slow cooker method only)
low-calorie cooking spray
500g stewing beef (all visible fat removed), diced
1 onion, diced
6 shallots, peeled and halved lengthways
2 garlic cloves, finely chopped
1 tbsp red wine vinegar
2 medium carrots, peeled and chopped
200g button mushrooms
2 tbsp tomato puree
1 bay leaf
250g potatoes, peeled and 125g thinly sliced, 125g cut into large dice

OVEN METHOD
🍲 **2 HOURS 10 MINS**

Preheat the oven to 160°C (fan 140°/gas mark 3) and make up the stock with the stock cubes and 500ml boiling water.

Spray a large flameproof casserole dish (with a lid) with low-calorie cooking spray and place over a medium-high heat. Add the meat to the pan and brown on all sides, then set aside. (If you have a small frying pan you may need to do this in batches to avoid overcrowding the pan.)

Add some more low-calorie cooking spray to the dish and sauté the onion, shallots and garlic over a medium heat for 3–4 minutes, until they start to soften.

Return the meat to the pan and add the remaining ingredients. Bring to the boil, cover and cook in the oven for about 2 hours, stirring halfway through. Remove the bay leaf and serve.

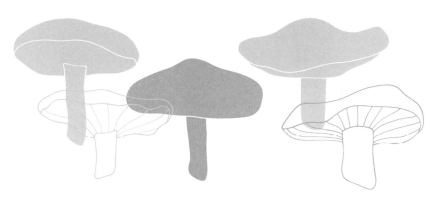

SLOW COOKER METHOD

🍲 4–6 HOURS

Make up the stock using the stock cubes, stock pot and 200ml boiling water.

Set the slow cooker to Sauté, spray it with some low-calorie cooking spray, add the meat, onion, shallots and garlic, and sauté until the meat is browned and the onions have softened.

If your slow cooker doesn't have a Sauté function, spray a large frying pan with low-calorie cooking spray and place over a medium-high heat. Add the meat to the pan and brown on all sides. (If you have a small frying pan you may need to do this in batches to avoid overcrowding the pan.) Place in the slow cooker.

Add some more low-calorie cooking spray to the frying pan and sauté the onion, shallots and garlic over a medium heat for 3–4 minutes until they start to soften. Add them to the slow cooker.

FOR A COLOUR IMAGE OF THIS RECIPE, PLEASE VISIT PINCHOFNOM.COM /PLANNER

Add the remaining ingredients (adding the extra stock pot), stir well, replace the lid and cook for 4 hours on High setting or 5–6 hours on Medium setting. When the meat is tender, stir (this will break up the potato and thicken the casserole). Remove the bay leaf and serve.

Week Seven

CHANGE +/-

CURRENT WEIGHT

THIS WEEK I WOULD LIKE TO ACHIEVE

LAST WEEK, THESE THINGS WENT WELL...

REMINDERS FOR THIS WEEK

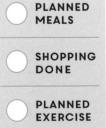

○ PLANNED
MEALS

○ SHOPPING
DONE

○ PLANNED
EXERCISE

IMAGINE
WHAT COULD
HAPPEN IF
YOU DON'T
GIVE UP

Day One

BREAKFAST

LUNCH

DINNER

SNACK 1

SNACK 2

TREATS

WATER

Day Two

BREAKFAST

LUNCH

DINNER

SNACK 1

SNACK 2

TREATS

WATER

WEEK 7

Day Three

BREAKFAST

LUNCH

DINNER

SNACK 1

SNACK 2

TREATS

WATER

74

Day Four

BREAKFAST

LUNCH

DINNER

SNACK 1

SNACK 2

TREATS

WATER

Day Five

BREAKFAST

LUNCH

DINNER

SNACK 1

SNACK 2

TREATS

WATER

Day Six

BREAKFAST

LUNCH

DINNER

SNACK 1

SNACK 2

TREATS

WATER

Day Seven

BREAKFAST

LUNCH

DINNER

SNACK 1

SNACK 2

TREATS

◐ ◐ ◐ ◐ ◐ ◐ ◐ ◐
◐ ◐ ◐ ◐ ◐ ◐ ◐

WATER

◇ ◇ ◇ ◇
◇ ◇ ◇ ◇

ROASTED VEGETABLE *and* BULGUR WHEAT SALAD

FOR A COLOUR IMAGE OF THIS RECIPE, PLEASE VISIT PINCHOFNOM.COM /PLANNER

🕐 **10 MINS** | 🍲 **30 MINS** | 🔥 **116 KCAL** PER SERVING

Bulgur wheat is found in many Middle Eastern dishes. It's higher in fibre than most whole grains and slightly lower in calories than other grains, such as brown rice. This salad has lovely Mediterranean flavours. It's perfect for making in bulk to refrigerate and snack on over a few days – simply hold back the herbs and stir through just before serving.

Everyday Light

V

SERVES 4

1 red pepper, halved, deseeded and cut into 2cm (¾in) chunks

1 yellow pepper, halved, deseeded and cut into 2cm (¾in) chunks

1 courgette, cut into 2cm (¾in) chunks

3 garlic cloves, peeled

200g carrots, cut into 1cm (½in)-thick slices

1 red onion, cut into wedges

low-calorie cooking spray

sea salt and freshly ground black pepper

250g bulgur wheat

1 vegetable stock cube

decent handful of fresh mint leaves

decent handful of flat-leaf parsley

decent handful of basil leaves

juice of 1 lemon

Preheat the oven to 200°C (fan 180°/gas mark 6).

Place the pepper, courgette, garlic, carrots and onion wedges on a large baking tray, spray liberally with low-calorie cooking spray, season with salt and pepper and roast in the oven for 25–30 minutes, or until the vegetables are soft and beginning to colour around the edges.

Meanwhile, place the bulgur wheat, stock cube and 1 litre of water in a large saucepan, bring to the boil, then reduce the heat and simmer for 15 minutes. Drain and return the bulgur wheat to the pan. Cover with a lid and allow to stand. It will finish cooking in its steam.

Roughly chop the fresh herbs.

When the vegetables are cooked, remove the garlic from the tray and mash it with the back of a fork.

Fluff up the bulgur wheat, then stir in the roasted vegetables, chopped herbs and lemon juice. Season to taste and serve.

Week Eight

CHANGE +/-

CURRENT WEIGHT

THIS WEEK I WOULD LIKE TO ACHIEVE

LAST WEEK, THESE THINGS WENT WELL...

REMINDERS FOR THIS WEEK

○ **PLANNED MEALS**

○ **SHOPPING DONE**

○ **PLANNED EXERCISE**

Day One

BREAKFAST

LUNCH

DINNER

SNACK 1

SNACK 2

TREATS

◐ ◐ ◐ ◐ ◐ ◐ ◐ ◐

◐ ◐ ◐ ◐ ◐ ◐ ◐

WATER

◇ ◇ ◇ ◇

◇ ◇ ◇ ◇

Day Two

BREAKFAST

LUNCH

DINNER

SNACK 1

SNACK 2

TREATS

WATER

Day Three

BREAKFAST

LUNCH

DINNER

SNACK 1

SNACK 2

TREATS

WATER

Day Four

BREAKFAST

LUNCH

DINNER

SNACK 1

SNACK 2

TREATS

WATER

Day Five

BREAKFAST

LUNCH

DINNER

SNACK 1

SNACK 2

TREATS

WATER

Day Six

BREAKFAST

LUNCH

DINNER

SNACK 1

SNACK 2

TREATS

WATER

Day Seven

BREAKFAST

LUNCH

DINNER

SNACK 1

SNACK 2

TREATS

WATER

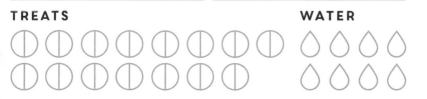

CHICKEN SAGWALA

🕐 **15 MINS** | 🍲 **30 MINS** | 🔥 **266 KCAL** PER SERVING

A sagwala is a spinach-based curry dish from India. This recipe uses a curry paste that you can make in advance and freeze, so you can make a quick curry any day of the week. Rich and flavoursome, you'll never need to order from the local Indian takeaway again.

Everyday Light

use GF stock cubes

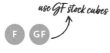

SERVES 4

low-calorie cooking spray
500g chicken breast (skin and
    visible fat removed), diced
1 onion, thickly sliced
1 red pepper, deseeded and
    thickly sliced
1 tsp garam masala
1 x 400g tin chopped
    tomatoes
150ml chicken stock
    (1 x chicken stock cube
    dissolved in 150ml
    boiling water)
200g spinach leaves
bunch of coriander (enough to
    lightly pack 1 cup), chopped

FOR THE CURRY PASTE

low-calorie cooking spray
1 fresh red chilli, halved
    lengthways, deseeded and
    roughly chopped
1 onion, chopped
2 garlic cloves, grated

First, make the curry paste. Spray a large frying pan or wok with low-calorie cooking spray and place over a medium heat. Add the chilli, onion, garlic and ginger and sauté until the onion begins to soften. Transfer to a food processor or blender, add the tomato puree and the spices, salt and pepper and blitz to a paste.

Give the frying pan or wok another good spray with low-calorie cooking spray and return to a medium heat.

Toss the diced chicken in a bowl with the curry paste until it is well coated, then add to the pan or wok. Fry gently for 3–4 minutes, then add the sliced onion and pepper, and the garam masala. Continue to cook for 3–4 minutes, then add the tinned tomatoes and chicken stock to the pan. Turn up the heat and bring the curry to the boil, then reduce the heat and allow it to simmer for 10 minutes.

Test the chicken to make sure it is cooked – there should be no pink in the middle. Add the spinach and keep stirring for a minute or two until the spinach wilts.

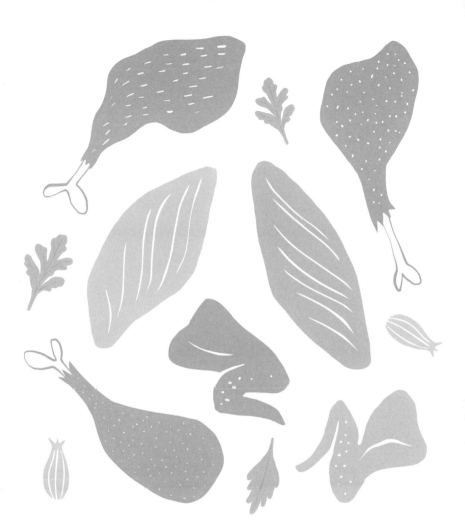

2cm (¾in) piece of root
   ginger, peeled and grated
1 tbsp tomato puree
1 tbsp smoked paprika
1 tsp ground cumin
1 tsp ground coriander
1 tsp ground cinnamon
1 tsp salt
½ tsp ground black pepper

Throw in the chopped coriander, stir, then remove
from the heat and serve with your choice of side dish.

FOR A
COLOUR IMAGE
OF THIS RECIPE,
PLEASE VISIT
PINCHOFNOM.COM
/PLANNER

Week Nine

CHANGE +/-

CURRENT WEIGHT

THIS WEEK I WOULD LIKE TO ACHIEVE

LAST WEEK, THESE THINGS WENT WELL...

REMINDERS FOR THIS WEEK

○ **PLANNED MEALS**

○ **SHOPPING DONE**

○ **PLANNED EXERCISE**

Day One

BREAKFAST

LUNCH

DINNER

SNACK 1

SNACK 2

TREATS

WATER

Day Two

BREAKFAST

LUNCH

DINNER

SNACK 1

SNACK 2

TREATS

WATER

Day Three

BREAKFAST

LUNCH

DINNER

SNACK 1

SNACK 2

TREATS

WATER

Day Four

BREAKFAST

LUNCH

DINNER

SNACK 1

SNACK 2

TREATS

WATER

Day Five

BREAKFAST

LUNCH

DINNER

SNACK 1

SNACK 2

TREATS

WATER

Day Six

BREAKFAST

LUNCH

DINNER

SNACK 1

SNACK 2

TREATS

WATER

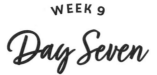

WEEK 9

Day Seven

BREAKFAST

LUNCH

DINNER

SNACK 1

SNACK 2

TREATS

WATER

Week Ten

CHANGE +/-

CURRENT WEIGHT

THIS WEEK I WOULD LIKE TO ACHIEVE

LAST WEEK, THESE THINGS WENT WELL...

REMINDERS FOR THIS WEEK

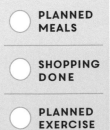

PLANNED
MEALS

SHOPPING
DONE

PLANNED
EXERCISE

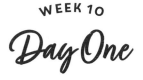

Day One

BREAKFAST

LUNCH

DINNER

SNACK 1

SNACK 2

TREATS

◯ ◯ ◯ ◯ ◯ ◯ ◯ ◯
◯ ◯ ◯ ◯ ◯ ◯ ◯ ◯

WATER

◇ ◇ ◇ ◇
◇ ◇ ◇ ◇

WEEK 10

Day Two

BREAKFAST

LUNCH

DINNER

SNACK 1

SNACK 2

TREATS

WATER

Day Three

BREAKFAST

LUNCH

DINNER

SNACK 1

SNACK 2

TREATS

WATER

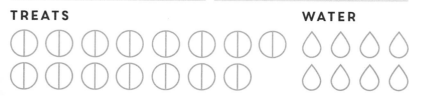

Day Four

BREAKFAST

LUNCH

DINNER

SNACK 1

SNACK 2

TREATS

WATER

Day Five

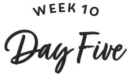

BREAKFAST

LUNCH

DINNER

SNACK 1

SNACK 2

TREATS

⊘ ⊘ ⊘ ⊘ ⊘ ⊘ ⊘ ⊘
⊘ ⊘ ⊘ ⊘ ⊘ ⊘ ⊘

WATER

◊ ◊ ◊ ◊
◊ ◊ ◊ ◊

Day Six

BREAKFAST

LUNCH

DINNER

SNACK 1

SNACK 2

TREATS

WATER

Day Seven

BREAKFAST

LUNCH

DINNER

SNACK 1

SNACK 2

TREATS

WATER

YOUVETSI

⏱ **10 MINS** | 🍲 **VARIABLE** SEE BELOW | 🔥 **535 KCAL** PER SERVING

Youvetsi is a gently spiced, baked Greek meat dish made with tomatoes. The rounded flavour of cinnamon cut through and balanced by the salty feta cheese makes this dish an absolute winner. Now there's no need to travel all the way to Greece to taste it!

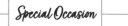

Special Occasion

F

SERVES 4

low-calorie cooking spray
500g stewing beef (visible fat removed), diced
1½ tsp dried oregano
½- tsp ground cinnamon
2 onions, sliced
2 tbsp red wine vinegar
1 bay leaf
sea salt and freshly ground black pepper
1 x 400g tin chopped tomatoes
1 litre beef stock (2 beef stock cubes and 1 beef stock pot dissolved in 1 litre boiling water)
2 tbsp tomato puree
400g orzo
130g reduced-fat feta cheese, crumbled

OVEN METHOD
🍲 **2 HOURS**

Preheat the oven to 180°C (fan 160°/gas mark 4).

Spray the casserole dish with low-calorie cooking spray. Add the beef, oregano, ground cinnamon, onions, red wine vinegar, bay leaf and plenty of salt and pepper and stir well. Bake in the oven, uncovered, for 20 minutes then stir.

Pour the chopped tomatoes into the dish, then the stock and tomato puree, cover tightly and return to the oven for 1½ hours until the beef is tender.

Remove the bay leaf, stir in the orzo, cover again and return to the oven for a further 20 minutes, stirring halfway through, until the orzo is cooked and the sauce has thickened.

Sprinkle with the crumbled feta and serve.

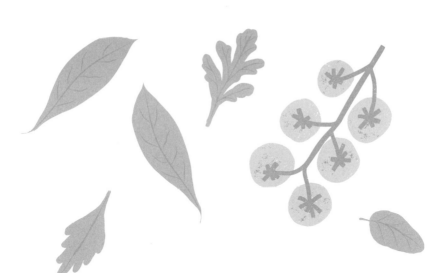

SLOW COOKER METHOD

🍲 **5–6 HOURS**

Spray a large frying pan with low-calorie cooking spray and place over a high heat. Add the beef, oregano, and ground cinnamon, season well with plenty of salt and pepper and cook for around 5 minutes until the beef has browned.

Tip the beef into the slow cooker, then add the onions, red wine vinegar, bay leaf, chopped tomatoes, stock and tomato puree and stir well. Set the slow cooker to High, cover and cook for 5–6 hours until the beef is tender.

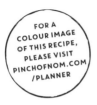

FOR A COLOUR IMAGE OF THIS RECIPE, PLEASE VISIT PINCHOFNOM.COM /PLANNER

Remove the bay leaf, stir in the orzo and cook for a further 20 minutes, stirring halfway through, until the orzo is cooked and the sauce has thickened.

Sprinkle with the crumbled feta and serve.

Week Eleven

CHANGE +/-

CURRENT WEIGHT

THIS WEEK I WOULD LIKE TO ACHIEVE

LAST WEEK, THESE THINGS WENT WELL...

REMINDERS FOR THIS WEEK

○ **PLANNED MEALS**

○ **SHOPPING DONE**

○ **PLANNED EXERCISE**

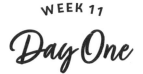

Day One

BREAKFAST

LUNCH

DINNER

SNACK 1

SNACK 2

TREATS

WATER

Day Two

BREAKFAST

LUNCH

DINNER

SNACK 1

SNACK 2

TREATS

WATER

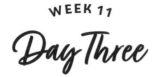

BREAKFAST

LUNCH

DINNER

SNACK 1

SNACK 2

TREATS

WATER

Day Four

BREAKFAST

LUNCH

DINNER

SNACK 1

SNACK 2

TREATS

WATER

Day Five

BREAKFAST

LUNCH

DINNER

SNACK 1

SNACK 2

TREATS

WATER

Day Six

BREAKFAST

LUNCH

DINNER

SNACK 1

SNACK 2

TREATS

WATER

Day Seven

BREAKFAST

LUNCH

DINNER

SNACK 1

SNACK 2

TREATS

WATER

TOMATO *and* CHILLI RISOTTO

⏱ **10 MINS** | 🍲 **45 MINS** | 🔥 **428 KCAL** PER SERVING

Risotto is one of those dishes that deserves the time and attention that goes into the process of making it. It's a real labour of love and you won't mind making this delicious, spicy version – rich with stock and tomatoes, while packing a little chilli punch – again and again.

Everyday Light

use GF stock pots

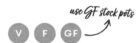

(V) (F) (GF)

SERVES 4

500g cherry tomatoes, halved
2 red peppers, deseeded and chopped
1–2 red chillies, deseeded and chopped
2 tbsp balsamic vinegar
1 tsp smoked paprika
sea salt and freshly ground black pepper
low-calorie cooking spray
2 onions, very finely chopped
4 garlic cloves, chopped
350g Arborio rice
1.5 litres vegetable stock (2 vegetable stock pots and 1 white wine stock pot dissolved in 1.5 litres boiling water)
small bunch of fresh basil

Preheat the oven to 200°C (fan 180°/gas mark 6).

Place the cherry tomatoes on a baking tray with the chopped red peppers and chillies, balsamic vinegar and paprika. Season with salt and pepper, and spray with a liberal coating of low-calorie cooking spray. Place the baking tray in the oven and roast for 40 minutes.

While the tomatoes, peppers and chillies are roasting, spray a large frying pan with some low-calorie cooking spray and place over a high heat. Add the onion and garlic and fry for about 5 minutes until the onions begin to brown, then turn down to a medium heat. Add the risotto rice to the onions and fry gently for about 5 minutes until the rice starts to turn translucent.

Add a couple of ladles of warm stock to the pan and stir until the liquid has been absorbed. Keep adding ladles of stock, a couple at a time, stirring until the liquid has absorbed between each addition and cook until the rice is tender, but still has a slight bite. This could take up to 40 minutes. Don't worry if you have stock left over – just use as much as you need until the rice is cooked.

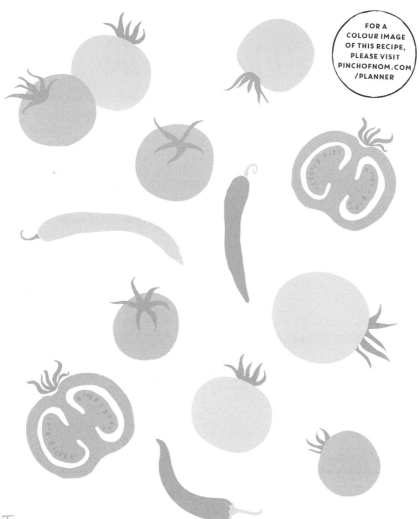

FOR A COLOUR IMAGE OF THIS RECIPE, PLEASE VISIT PINCHOFNOM.COM /PLANNER

Tip

IF YOU HAVEN'T GOT A JUG BIG ENOUGH TO MAKE UP 1.5 LITRES OF STOCK, MAKE THE STOCK UP IN A LARGE SAUCEPAN OR MAKE IT UP IN 500ML BATCHES, USING ONE STOCK POT IN EACH BATCH.

When the rice is ready, take the pan off the heat.

Take the roasted tomato and pepper mixture out of the oven and mix it into the rice. Tear up a handful of basil leaves and stir them into the risotto. Season to taste with salt and pepper and serve.

Week Twelve

CHANGE +/-

CURRENT WEIGHT

THIS WEEK I WOULD LIKE TO ACHIEVE

LAST WEEK, THESE THINGS WENT WELL...

REMINDERS FOR THIS WEEK

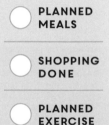

◯ **PLANNED MEALS**

◯ **SHOPPING DONE**

◯ **PLANNED EXERCISE**

Believe

YOU CAN

&

YOU WILL

Day One

BREAKFAST

LUNCH

DINNER

SNACK 1

SNACK 2

TREATS

WATER

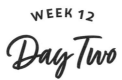

Day Two

BREAKFAST

LUNCH

DINNER

SNACK 1

SNACK 2

TREATS

WATER

Day Three

BREAKFAST

LUNCH

DINNER

SNACK 1

SNACK 2

TREATS

WATER

Day Four

BREAKFAST

LUNCH

DINNER

SNACK 1

SNACK 2

TREATS

WATER

Day Five

BREAKFAST

LUNCH

DINNER

SNACK 1

SNACK 2

TREATS

WATER

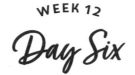

Day Six

BREAKFAST

LUNCH

DINNER

SNACK 1

SNACK 2

TREATS

WATER

Day Seven

BREAKFAST

LUNCH

DINNER

SNACK 1

SNACK 2

TREATS

WATER

CHOUX BUNS

🕐 **20 MINS** | 🍲 **45 MINS** PLUS COOLING | 🔥 **102 KCAL** PER SERVING

Choux pastry can't possibly be something you can enjoy while losing weight, right? Wrong! A few simple substitutions for lower-calorie counterparts and you won't believe the amazing taste and authenticity of these choux buns. You could even drizzle with a bit of melted dark chocolate – just remember to add this to the calorie count if you do!

--- *Special Occasion* ---

Buns only

F

MAKES 10 BUNS

100g reduced-fat spread
1 tsp granulated sweetener
pinch of salt
100g self-raising flour
2 large eggs
20 tbsp reduced-fat
  aerosol cream
1 tsp icing sugar

FOR A COLOUR IMAGE OF THIS RECIPE, PLEASE VISIT PINCHOFNOM.COM /PLANNER

Preheat the oven to 180°C (fan 160°/gas mark 4) and line a baking tray with greaseproof paper.

Put the reduced-fat spread, sweetener, salt and 150ml water in a saucepan and bring to the boil, then remove from the heat and stir in the flour – it will look lumpy to start with but don't worry, just keep stirring! Once the mixture starts to form a ball, add one of the eggs. Beat until glossy then add the next egg. The mixture looks like it is going to separate but with elbow grease it combines to a silky batter.

Spoon the choux mixture into a piping bag with a large star (or plain) nozzle attachment and pipe ten buns onto the lined baking tray. Tap down the 'tails' on the top of the buns with a wet finger and place in the oven for 35 minutes. DO NOT OPEN THE DOOR!

After 35 minutes, turn the buns over and return to the oven for another 10 minutes.

Remove from the oven and leave the buns to cool completely. (You can freeze them at this point, prior to filling.) When cooled, cut them in half, squirt in about 2 tablespoons of the cream, dust with icing sugar and serve immediately.

Week Thirteen

CHANGE +/-

CURRENT WEIGHT

THIS WEEK I WOULD LIKE TO ACHIEVE

LAST WEEK, THESE THINGS WENT WELL...

REMINDERS FOR THIS WEEK

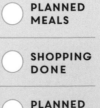

○ PLANNED MEALS

○ SHOPPING DONE

○ PLANNED EXERCISE

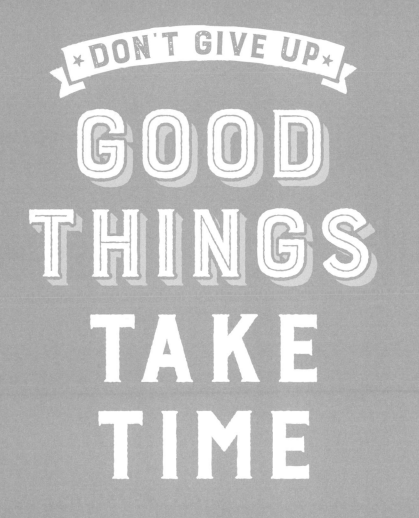

Day One

BREAKFAST

LUNCH

DINNER

SNACK 1

SNACK 2

TREATS

WATER

Day Two

BREAKFAST

LUNCH

DINNER

SNACK 1

SNACK 2

TREATS

WATER

Day Three

BREAKFAST

LUNCH

DINNER

SNACK 1

SNACK 2

TREATS

WATER

Day Four

BREAKFAST

LUNCH

DINNER

SNACK 1

SNACK 2

TREATS

WATER

Day Five

BREAKFAST

LUNCH

DINNER

SNACK 1

SNACK 2

TREATS

WATER

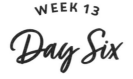

Day Six

BREAKFAST

LUNCH

DINNER

SNACK 1

SNACK 2

TREATS

WATER

Day Seven

BREAKFAST

LUNCH

DINNER

SNACK 1

SNACK 2

TREATS

WATER

BACON *and* CHIVE EGGY BREAD

FOR A COLOUR IMAGE OF THIS RECIPE, PLEASE VISIT PINCHOFNOM.COM /PLANNER

🕐 **5 MINS** | 🍲 **8 MINS** | 🔥 **308 KCAL** PER SERVING

The secret to good eggy bread is to let the bread sit in the egg and really soak it all up – you don't want scrambled egg either side of bread: you want moist, rich, springy eggy-bread deliciousness with salty bacon and a pinch of chopped chives to brighten up your morning. Mmmm, heaven!

Weekly Indulgence

SERVES 1

low-calorie cooking spray
2 bacon medallions
2 medium eggs
small bunch of fresh chives, chopped
1 tsp Worcestershire sauce
sea salt and freshly ground black pepper
2 slices of wholemeal bread (small slices, 60g in total)

Tip

IF YOU ARE MAKING THIS FOR MORE THAN ONE PERSON, PREHEAT THE OVEN TO A LOW TEMPERATURE AND KEEP THE COOKED EGGY BREAD WARM BETWEEN BATCHES.

Spray a frying pan with some low-calorie cooking spray, add the bacon medallions and fry until cooked, then remove from the heat and set to one side.

Whisk the eggs in a wide, shallow bowl. Add most of the chopped chives (setting some aside for later) and the Worcestershire sauce and season with salt and pepper.

Chop the cooked bacon into little pieces and add to the egg mix.

Dip the bread slices into the egg mix, turning the bread to allow the egg mix to soak into both sides of the bread.

Spray the frying pan with some more low-calorie cooking spray and place it over a low–medium heat. Cook the eggy bread for 2–4 minutes on each side. It should be golden but be careful not to burn it.

Serve the eggy bread with the rest of the chopped fresh chives scattered on top.

Week Fourteen

CHANGE +/-

CURRENT WEIGHT

THIS WEEK I WOULD LIKE TO ACHIEVE

LAST WEEK, THESE THINGS WENT WELL...

REMINDERS FOR THIS WEEK

○ **PLANNED MEALS**

○ **SHOPPING DONE**

○ **PLANNED EXERCISE**

Day One

BREAKFAST

LUNCH

DINNER

SNACK 1

SNACK 2

TREATS

WATER

Day Two

BREAKFAST

LUNCH

DINNER

SNACK 1

SNACK 2

TREATS

WATER

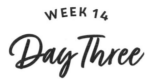

Day Three

BREAKFAST

LUNCH

DINNER

SNACK 1

SNACK 2

TREATS

WATER

Day Four

BREAKFAST

LUNCH

DINNER

SNACK 1

SNACK 2

TREATS

WATER

Day Five

BREAKFAST

LUNCH

DINNER

SNACK 1

SNACK 2

TREATS

WATER

Day Six

BREAKFAST

LUNCH

DINNER

SNACK 1

SNACK 2

TREATS

WATER

Day Seven

BREAKFAST

LUNCH

DINNER

SNACK 1

SNACK 2

TREATS

WATER

MEXICAN *chilli* PIE

🕐 **10 MINS** | 🍲 **1 HOUR 20 MINS** | 🔥 **307 KCAL** PER SERVING

Those shepherds have had a pie for centuries without anyone daring to mess with it. Pinch of Nom decided to mess with the shepherds! We added some Mexican flavours to this popular, traditionally British dish and came up with something extraordinary. With added spice, pepper and beans, this recipe transforms into something else entirely and is sure to become a family favourite.

Everyday Light

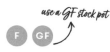

use a GF stock pot

F **GF**

SERVES 8

low-calorie cooking spray
500g 5%-fat minced beef
1 courgette, chopped into 1cm
   (½in) dice
1 large red pepper, deseeded
   and chopped into
   1cm (½in) pieces
2 garlic cloves, crushed
1 onion, roughly chopped
2 tbsp tomato puree
1 tbsp ground cumin
1–2 tsp chilli powder
pinch of dried chilli flakes
1 tsp dried oregano
390g tomato passata
1 x 400g tin chopped tomatoes
200g tinned sweetcorn, drained
1 x 390g tin mixed beans in
   chilli sauce (or 1 x 390g tin
   kidney beans in chilli sauce)
1 beef stock pot

Spray a saucepan with low-calorie cooking spray and place over a medium heat. Add the mince and fry until browned, breaking up the mince with a wooden spoon, then add the courgette, pepper, garlic and onion and cook for about 5 minutes until the vegetables start to soften. Stir in the tomato puree, cumin, chilli powder (to taste) and chilli flakes, mix and cook for another couple of minutes.

Add all of the other ingredients (except the potatoes), season to taste and leave to simmer over a low heat for 40 minutes.

Meanwhile, make the mashed potato topping by bringing a large saucepan of salted water to the boil. Add the potatoes and cook for 10–15 minutes until the potatoes are tender. Drain and mash until smooth and fluffy and preheat the oven to 180°C (fan 160°/gas mark 4).

When the chilli mix has finished simmering, transfer it to a large, ovenproof dish. If you find there is too much liquid in the chilli mix, turn the heat up until

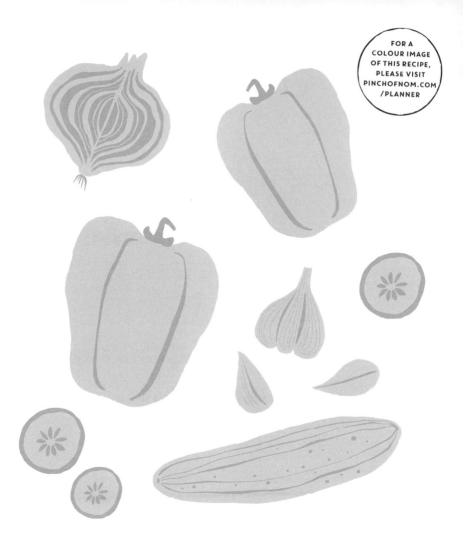

FOR A COLOUR IMAGE OF THIS RECIPE, PLEASE VISIT PINCHOFNOM.COM /PLANNER

sea salt and freshly ground
black pepper
1kg potatoes, peeled and
quartered

the sauce is bubbling (stirring frequently to avoid it
catching at the bottom) and let it reduce a little.
Top the chilli mix with the mashed potato and
roughen the surface with a fork.

Bake in the oven for about 40 minutes until the top is
crisp and golden. Remove from the oven and serve.

Week Fifteen

CHANGE +/-

CURRENT WEIGHT

THIS WEEK I WOULD LIKE TO ACHIEVE

LAST WEEK, THESE THINGS WENT WELL...

REMINDERS FOR THIS WEEK

○ **PLANNED MEALS**

○ **SHOPPING DONE**

○ **PLANNED EXERCISE**

Day One

BREAKFAST

LUNCH

DINNER

SNACK 1

SNACK 2

TREATS

WATER

Day Two

BREAKFAST

LUNCH

DINNER

SNACK 1

SNACK 2

TREATS

WATER

Day Three

BREAKFAST

LUNCH

DINNER

SNACK 1

SNACK 2

TREATS

WATER

Day Four

BREAKFAST

LUNCH

DINNER

SNACK 1

SNACK 2

TREATS

WATER

Day Five

BREAKFAST

LUNCH

DINNER

SNACK 1

SNACK 2

TREATS

WATER

Day Six

BREAKFAST

LUNCH

DINNER

SNACK 1

SNACK 2

TREATS

WATER

Day Seven

BREAKFAST

LUNCH

DINNER

SNACK 1

SNACK 2

TREATS

WATER

Week Sixteen

CHANGE +/-

CURRENT WEIGHT

THIS WEEK I WOULD LIKE TO ACHIEVE

LAST WEEK, THESE THINGS WENT WELL...

REMINDERS FOR THIS WEEK

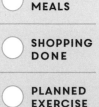

○ PLANNED MEALS

○ SHOPPING DONE

○ PLANNED EXERCISE

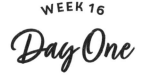

Day One

BREAKFAST

LUNCH

DINNER

SNACK 1

SNACK 2

TREATS

WATER

Day Two

BREAKFAST

LUNCH

DINNER

SNACK 1

SNACK 2

TREATS

WATER

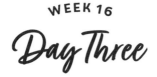

Day Three

BREAKFAST

LUNCH

DINNER

SNACK 1

SNACK 2

TREATS

WATER

Day Four

BREAKFAST

LUNCH

DINNER

SNACK 1

SNACK 2

TREATS

WATER

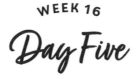

Day Five

BREAKFAST

LUNCH

DINNER

SNACK 1

SNACK 2

TREATS

◐ ◐ ◐ ◐ ◐ ◐ ◐ ◐
◐ ◐ ◐ ◐ ◐ ◐

WATER

◇ ◇ ◇ ◇
◇ ◇ ◇ ◇

Day Six

BREAKFAST

LUNCH

DINNER

SNACK 1

SNACK 2

TREATS

WATER

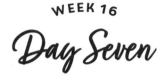

Day Seven

BREAKFAST

LUNCH

DINNER

SNACK 1

SNACK 2

TREATS

WATER

APPLE PUFFS

⏱ **20 MINS** | 🍲 **25 MINS** | 🔥 **34 KCAL** PER PUFF

These little apple puffs taste divine. Using a light puff pastry and a little sweetener in place of sugar, these sweet treats are calorie-friendly as well as taste-friendly. They are perfect for serving up to friends, or if you don't want them to disappear, hide them away and have a few moments of 'you time' without friends or family being any the wiser.

Special Occasion

(F)

MAKES 40 PUFFS

150g cooking apple
1 tbsp granulated sweetener
½ tsp mixed spice
½ tsp ground cinnamon
375g sheet light puff pastry
a little icing sugar, for dusting (optional)

Line a baking tray with greaseproof paper and preheat the oven to 160°C (fan 140°/gas mark 3).

Peel and slice the cooking apple into a saucepan, add the granulated sweetener, mixed spice, cinnamon and a splash of water and cook over a low heat for about 15 minutes until the apple has completely broken down. You may need to add an extra splash of water if the mixture starts to become dry and stick to the bottom, but don't add too much as you don't want the mixture to be runny! Remove from the heat and leave to cool for 10 minutes.

Meanwhile, place the rectangle of pastry on a clean surface with the long edge nearest you. Cut into four equal strips vertically, and then in half horizontally so you have eight pieces.

When the apple mixture has cooled, spread it over the pastry rectangles. Roll each rectangle from the short edge so you have 'Swiss rolls' of pastry and apple. Cut each pastry roll into five pieces – it will be quite soft, but cut straight down with a sharp knife; you can reshape them when they are on the baking tray and they will naturally bake into a spiral shape!

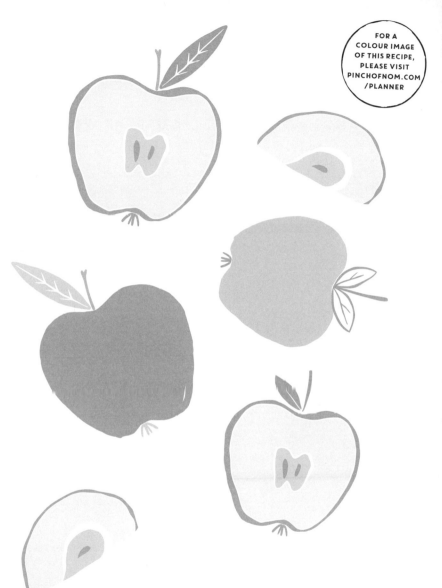

FOR A
COLOUR IMAGE
OF THIS RECIPE,
PLEASE VISIT
PINCHOFNOM.COM
/PLANNER

Place each puff on the lined baking tray and bake in the oven for 25 minutes until golden.

Remove from the oven, shake over a little icing sugar if desired, and serve.

Week Seventeen

CHANGE +/-

CURRENT WEIGHT

THIS WEEK I WOULD LIKE TO ACHIEVE

LAST WEEK, THESE THINGS WENT WELL...

REMINDERS FOR THIS WEEK

○ **PLANNED MEALS**

○ **SHOPPING DONE**

○ **PLANNED EXERCISE**

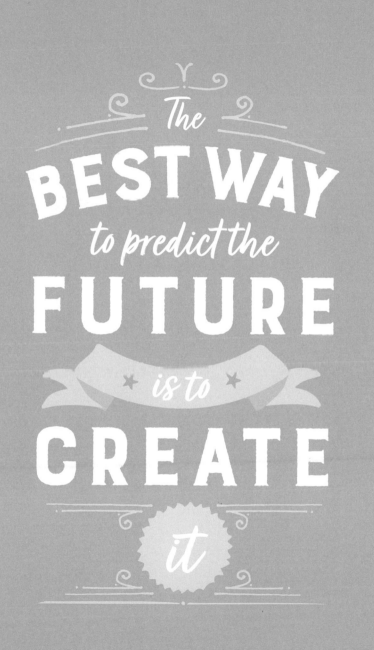

The
BEST WAY
to predict the
FUTURE
is to
CREATE
it

Day One

BREAKFAST

LUNCH

DINNER

SNACK 1

SNACK 2

TREATS

○ ○ ○ ○ ○ ○ ○ ○
○ ○ ○ ○ ○ ○ ○

WATER

◇ ◇ ◇ ◇
◇ ◇ ◇ ◇

Day Two

BREAKFAST

LUNCH

DINNER

SNACK 1

SNACK 2

TREATS

WATER

Day Three

BREAKFAST

LUNCH

DINNER

SNACK 1

SNACK 2

TREATS

◑ ◑ ◑ ◑ ◑ ◑ ◑ ◑
◑ ◑ ◑ ◑ ◑ ◑ ◑

WATER

◇ ◇ ◇ ◇
◇ ◇ ◇ ◇

Day Four

BREAKFAST

LUNCH

DINNER

SNACK 1

SNACK 2

TREATS

WATER

Day Five

BREAKFAST

LUNCH

DINNER

SNACK 1

SNACK 2

TREATS

WATER

Day Six

BREAKFAST

LUNCH

DINNER

SNACK 1

SNACK 2

TREATS

⊘ ⊘ ⊘ ⊘ ⊘ ⊘ ⊘ ⊘
⊘ ⊘ ⊘ ⊘ ⊘ ⊘ ⊘

WATER

◇ ◇ ◇ ◇
◇ ◇ ◇ ◇

Day Seven

BREAKFAST

LUNCH

DINNER

SNACK 1

SNACK 2

TREATS

WATER

SALT *and* PEPPER MUSHROOMS

FOR A COLOUR IMAGE OF THIS RECIPE, PLEASE VISIT PINCHOFNOM.COM /PLANNER

🕐 **10 MINS** | 🍲 **10 MINS** | 🔥 **46 KCAL** PER SERVING

Our salt and pepper seasoning is well loved by Pinch of Nom's online community. We've created salt and pepper chips, salt and pepper chicken and now … salt and pepper mushrooms. These work so well! They are such a perfect side dish or snack for when you feel like something that's naughty but really isn't!

Everyday Light

V **GF**

SERVES 4

low-calorie cooking spray
3 spring onions, trimmed and thinly sliced
½ red pepper, finely diced
½ green pepper, finely diced
½ red chilli, finely diced (use more if you like it fiery!)
600g mushrooms of choice, cut into large chunks (leave smaller ones whole)
1 tsp rice vinegar

FOR THE SPICE MIX

1 tbsp sea salt flakes
1 tbsp granulated sweetener
½ tbsp Chinese 5-spice
pinch of dried chilli flakes
½ tsp ground white pepper

Start by making the salt and pepper mix. Toast the sea salt in a frying pan until it starts to brown, then set aside to cool. Mix all the other ingredients together in a bowl, then add the cooled sea salt.

Spray a medium frying pan with some low-calorie cooking spray and place over a medium heat. Add the spring onions, peppers and chilli and fry for 3–4 minutes until soft, then set aside.

Spray the pan with a little more low-calorie cooking spray, then fry the mushrooms for 5–6 minutes until cooked, draining off any excess liquid that the mushrooms have released. Stir in the salt and pepper mix, peppers, spring onion and chilli, then add the rice vinegar and stir until it has evaporated.

Remove from the heat and serve.

Week Eighteen

CHANGE +/-

CURRENT WEIGHT

THIS WEEK I WOULD LIKE TO ACHIEVE

LAST WEEK, THESE THINGS WENT WELL...

REMINDERS FOR THIS WEEK

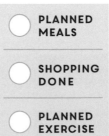

PLANNED MEALS

SHOPPING DONE

PLANNED EXERCISE

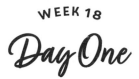

Day One

BREAKFAST

LUNCH

DINNER

SNACK 1

SNACK 2

TREATS

WATER

Day Two

BREAKFAST

LUNCH

DINNER

SNACK 1

SNACK 2

TREATS

WATER

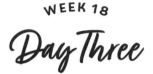

Day Three

BREAKFAST

LUNCH

DINNER

SNACK 1

SNACK 2

TREATS

WATER

Day Four

BREAKFAST

LUNCH

DINNER

SNACK 1

SNACK 2

TREATS

WATER

Day Five

BREAKFAST

LUNCH

DINNER

SNACK 1

SNACK 2

TREATS

WATER

Day Six

BREAKFAST

LUNCH

DINNER

SNACK 1

SNACK 2

TREATS

WATER

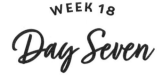

Day Seven

BREAKFAST

LUNCH

DINNER

SNACK 1

SNACK 2

TREATS

WATER

FOR COLOUR IMAGES OF THESE RECIPES, PLEASE VISIT PINCHOFNOM.COM /PLANNER

FRUIT SALAD 'PIZZA'

⏱ **10 MINS** | 🍲 **NO COOK** | 🔥 **88 KCAL** PER SERVING

Fruit … and pizza? Well, not quite. No heavy dough base to be found here, just refreshing watermelon. With loads of varieties of fruit on a creamy, delicious topping, it will feel more indulgent than real pizza, but without any of the guilt! Guilt-free 'pizza' is an idea we can 100% get behind!

Weekly Indulgence

V **GF**

SERVES 2

75g fat-free Greek-style yoghurt
1 tsp granulated sweetener
¼ tsp vanilla extract
1 large watermelon
10 blueberries
4 grapes
4 raspberries
4 strawberries
fresh mint leaves, to serve

Mix the yoghurt, sweetener and vanilla extract together in a bowl then set to one side.

Cut the watermelon in half, then cut a large slice from one side. This will be your 'pizza' base. You can pick out the seeds carefully from each side of the slice if you want to at this point.

Spread the yoghurt mix over the top of the slice.

Slice the remaining fruit into halves and thin slices and arrange on top of the watermelon. Slice the 'pizza' and serve with fresh mint leaves scattered on top.

Tip

YOU CAN TOP WITH YOUR FAVOURITE FRUITS OR WHATEVER YOU HAVE AVAILABLE.

CHIPOTLE SWEET POTATO HASSELBACKS

🕐 **10 MINS** | 🍲 **50 MINS–1 HOUR** | 💧 **131 KCAL** PER SERVING

Who doesn't love the smoky spice of chipotle? Adding it to the sweetness of sweet potato, this is such a simple recipe, but it bursts with flavour. One of our taste testers described this recipe as 'well fit'. We're taking that description and running with it. These chipotle sweet potato hasselbacks are well fit!

--- *Everyday Light* ---

SERVES 4

1 tbsp chipotle chilli flakes
1 tbsp smoked paprika
1 tbsp English mustard powder
1 tbsp ground cumin
2 tbsp granulated brown sweetener
1 tbsp salt
pinch of dried thyme
1 tbsp garlic granules
4 sweet potatoes
low-calorie cooking spray
green salad, to serve

Preheat the oven to 200°C fan (180°/gas mark 6).

Mix the spices, sweetener, salt, thyme and garlic granules together in a bowl.

Thinly slice the potatoes at roughly 5mm (¼ in) intervals, so you go about three-quarters of the way through the potato but it still holds together. Separate the slices slightly.

Spray the sweet potatoes with low-calorie cooking spray and rub about 1 tablespoon of spice mix into the inside slices of the potato.

Place the hasselbacks on a baking sheet and bake in the oven for 50 minutes–1 hour, depending on the size of the potatoes – they are cooked when you can easily insert a knife into them.

Remove from the oven and serve with a green salad.

Week Nineteen

CHANGE +/-

CURRENT WEIGHT

THIS WEEK I WOULD LIKE TO ACHIEVE

LAST WEEK, THESE THINGS WENT WELL...

REMINDERS FOR THIS WEEK

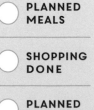

- ○ PLANNED MEALS
- ○ SHOPPING DONE
- ○ PLANNED EXERCISE

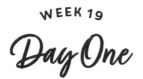

WEEK 19
Day One

BREAKFAST

LUNCH

DINNER

SNACK 1

SNACK 2

TREATS

WATER

Day Two

BREAKFAST

LUNCH

DINNER

SNACK 1

SNACK 2

TREATS

WATER

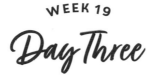

Day Three

BREAKFAST

LUNCH

DINNER

SNACK 1

SNACK 2

TREATS

○ ○ ○ ○ ○ ○ ○ ○
○ ○ ○ ○ ○ ○ ○

WATER

◇ ◇ ◇ ◇
◇ ◇ ◇ ◇

Day Four

BREAKFAST

LUNCH

DINNER

SNACK 1

SNACK 2

TREATS

WATER

Day Five

BREAKFAST

LUNCH

DINNER

SNACK 1

SNACK 2

TREATS

WATER

Day Six

BREAKFAST

LUNCH

DINNER

SNACK 1

SNACK 2

TREATS

WATER

Day Seven

BREAKFAST

LUNCH

DINNER

SNACK 1

SNACK 2

TREATS

WATER

Smoked
HADDOCK CHOWDER

🕐 **5 MINS** | 🍲 **20 MINS** | 🔥 **425 KCAL** PER SERVING

This dish, comprised of beautiful, flaked pieces of smoked haddock and a creamy chowder, is packed full of flavour. Fish is a great, protein-packed ingredient, which makes this chowder the perfect low-calorie, filling lunch.

―――――――――――――― *Weekly Indulgence* ――――――――――――――

SERVES 4

low-calorie cooking spray
1 large onion, roughly chopped
500g potatoes, peeled and
   cut into 2cm (¾ in) cubes
325g tinned sweetcorn, drained
700ml skimmed milk
sea salt and freshly ground
   black pepper
4 small smoked haddock
   fillets (skinless and boneless)
100g asparagus spears,
   trimmed and cut into
   3cm (1¼ in) lengths
2 tbsp fresh chopped chives

FOR A COLOUR IMAGE OF THIS RECIPE, PLEASE VISIT PINCHOFNOM.COM /PLANNER

Spray a large saucepan with some low-calorie cooking spray, place over a medium heat, add the onion and cook for a couple of minutes until softened.

Add the chopped potatoes to the saucepan with the onion, along with the drained sweetcorn, skimmed milk and 200ml water. Season with salt and pepper, being careful not to add too much salt as the fish is salty too. Bring to the boil then turn the heat down to a gentle simmer and cook for 5 minutes.

Add the smoked haddock fillets to the pan, making sure they are covered by the milk, and cook for a further 10 minutes, by which time the potatoes should be just starting to break up.

Meanwhile, cook the asparagus. Bring some water to the boil in a small saucepan, add the asparagus and cook for 2–3 minutes until just tender. Drain.

Using a slotted spoon, carefully remove the fish fillets from the pan, ensuring they don't break apart. Remove about a third of the potato, sweetcorn and onion mix, leaving the rest in the pan with the milk.

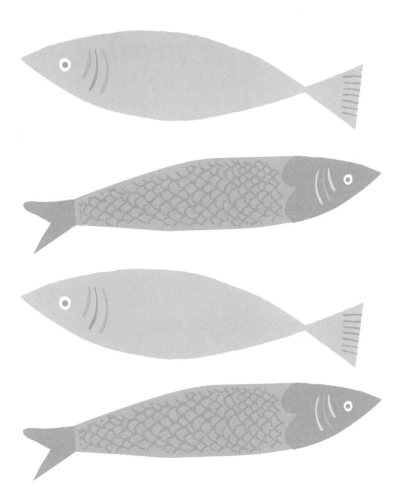

Blitz the milk mixture using a stick blender (or use a food processor) until smooth. Heat gently and add the potato, sweetcorn and onion mix that you set aside. Flake the fish in large chunks into the soup and add the chopped chives. Stir very carefully, making sure you don't break up the fish too much.

Serve warm, topped with the asparagus.

Week Twenty

CHANGE +/-

CURRENT WEIGHT

THIS WEEK I WOULD LIKE TO ACHIEVE

LAST WEEK, THESE THINGS WENT WELL...

REMINDERS FOR THIS WEEK

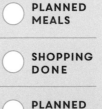

○ PLANNED MEALS

○ SHOPPING DONE

○ PLANNED EXERCISE

Day One

BREAKFAST

LUNCH

DINNER

SNACK 1

SNACK 2

TREATS

WATER

Day Two

BREAKFAST

LUNCH

DINNER

SNACK 1

SNACK 2

TREATS

WATER

Day Three

BREAKFAST

LUNCH

DINNER

SNACK 1

SNACK 2

TREATS

WATER

Day Four

BREAKFAST

LUNCH

DINNER

SNACK 1

SNACK 2

TREATS

WATER

Day Five

BREAKFAST

LUNCH

DINNER

SNACK 1

SNACK 2

TREATS

WATER

Day Six

BREAKFAST

LUNCH

DINNER

SNACK 1

SNACK 2

TREATS

WATER

Day Seven

BREAKFAST

LUNCH

DINNER

SNACK 1

SNACK 2

TREATS

⬭ ⬭ ⬭ ⬭ ⬭ ⬭ ⬭ ⬭

⬭ ⬭ ⬭ ⬭ ⬭ ⬭ ⬭

WATER

◊ ◊ ◊ ◊

◊ ◊ ◊ ◊

CHILLI 'PANEER'

⏱ **5 MINS** | 🍲 **35 MINS** | 🔥 **107 KCAL** PER SERVING

This 'paneer' recipe doesn't actually use paneer. Crazy, we know! But trust us ... you won't know it. Paneer is an Indian cheese with a firm texture and light taste. By substituting extra-firm, ready-pressed tofu for the paneer, you can recreate the taste and texture but drastically reduce the fat and calories. Serve as a side dish or double up the portion size for a quick and tasty main. This is a spicy dish, but reduce the chilli if you prefer it cooler.

Everyday Light

**SERVES 4
(AS A SIDE DISH)**

280g extra-firm tofu, cut into
   small cubes
2 tbsp soy sauce
1 tbsp garlic granules
1 tbsp onion granules
2 tbsp chilli powder
1 tsp granulated sweetener
2 tbsp lime juice
3 garlic cloves, finely chopped
1 tbsp dried chilli flakes
1 vegetable stock cube
1 large onion, finely chopped
low-calorie cooking spray
handful of fresh coriander
   (optional)

Preheat the oven to 220°C (fan 200°/gas mark 7).

Put the tofu in a bowl with the soy sauce, garlic granules, onion granules, chilli powder, sweetener and lime juice. Mix to coat the tofu and set to one side.

Put the garlic in a frying pan with the chilli flakes, then crumble in the stock cube and add 50ml water. Fry lightly over low–medium heat to release the aromatics, being careful not to burn the garlic. You should be left with a fragrant paste.

Add the chopped onion to the pan with another 50ml water and fry for a few minutes in the spices.

Spray the tofu in the bowl with some low-calorie cooking spray and add to the pan of onions. Fry for a few minutes.

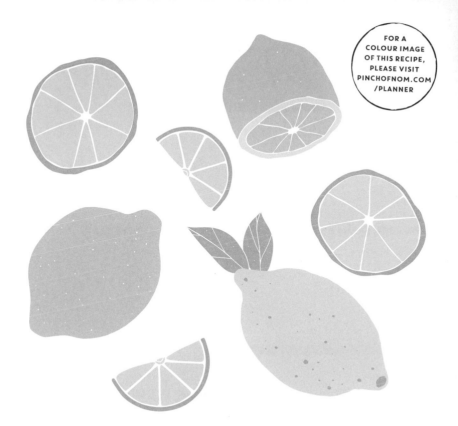

FOR A COLOUR IMAGE OF THIS RECIPE, PLEASE VISIT PINCHOFNOM.COM /PLANNER

Tip

LIME JUICE IS AVAILABLE FROM THE SUPERMARKET IN BOTTLES – YOU DON'T HAVE TO USE FRESH! IF YOU DON'T HAVE LIME JUICE, SUBSTITUTE WITH LEMON JUICE.

Spray a medium ovenproof dish with more low-calorie cooking spray and transfer the contents of the frying pan into it. Bake in the middle of the oven for 15 minutes, then turn the tofu and bake for another 15 minutes.

Remove from the oven and serve, scattered with fresh coriander if you like.

Week Twenty-One

CHANGE +/-

CURRENT WEIGHT

THIS WEEK I WOULD LIKE TO ACHIEVE

LAST WEEK, THESE THINGS WENT WELL...

REMINDERS FOR THIS WEEK

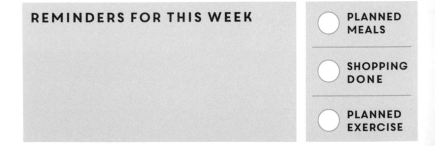

○ PLANNED MEALS

○ SHOPPING DONE

○ PLANNED EXERCISE

Don't RUIN A GOOD TODAY BECAUSE OF A BAD YESTERDAY

Day One

BREAKFAST

LUNCH

DINNER

SNACK 1

SNACK 2

TREATS

WATER

Day Two

BREAKFAST

LUNCH

DINNER

SNACK 1

SNACK 2

TREATS

WATER

Day Three

BREAKFAST

LUNCH

DINNER

SNACK 1

SNACK 2

TREATS

WATER

Day Four

BREAKFAST

LUNCH

DINNER

SNACK 1

SNACK 2

TREATS

WATER

Day Five

BREAKFAST

LUNCH

DINNER

SNACK 1

SNACK 2

TREATS

WATER

Day Six

BREAKFAST

LUNCH

DINNER

SNACK 1

SNACK 2

TREATS

WATER

Day Seven

BREAKFAST

LUNCH

DINNER

SNACK 1

SNACK 2

TREATS

WATER

ELDERFLOWER SPRITZ

🕙 **10 MINS** | 🍲 **NO COOK** | 🔥 **6 KCAL** PER SERVING

If there's an evening in those warm months of summer that doesn't involve a spritz, we don't want to know about it! This version is alcohol-free, to save on the calories, but you can always add a dash of a spirit if you'd prefer to spend a few calories on a boozy version. Perfectly balanced with elderflower, green tea and mint, this spritz is sure to become a summertime favourite.

Special Occasion

SERVES 4

1 x green tea bag
200ml boiling water
large handful of ice cubes
50ml sugar-free elderflower
  cordial
2 slices of cucumber
handful of fresh mint leaves
juice of 1 lemon
1 litre slimline tonic water
cucumber and lemon
  slices, to serve (optional)

Brew the green tea bag with the boiling water in a mug.

Once the tea has cooled, remove the tea bag and add the tea to a cocktail shaker with ice, the elderflower cordial, the 2 slices of cucumber, mint leaves and the lemon juice. Cover and shake thoroughly.

Strain the mix into glasses and top up with the slimline tonic. Garnish (if you wish) and serve.

Tip

IF YOU WANT TO MAKE IT ALCOHOLIC, A SHOT OF VODKA OR GIN WOULD WORK REALLY WELL WITH THESE FLAVOURS.

FOR A COLOUR IMAGE OF THIS RECIPE, PLEASE VISIT PINCHOFNOM.COM /PLANNER

Week Twenty-Two

CHANGE +/-

CURRENT WEIGHT

THIS WEEK I WOULD LIKE TO ACHIEVE

LAST WEEK, THESE THINGS WENT WELL...

REMINDERS FOR THIS WEEK

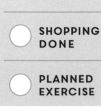

○ PLANNED MEALS

○ SHOPPING DONE

○ PLANNED EXERCISE

Day One

BREAKFAST

LUNCH

DINNER

SNACK 1

SNACK 2

TREATS

WATER

Day Two

BREAKFAST

LUNCH

DINNER

SNACK 1

SNACK 2

TREATS

WATER

Day Three

BREAKFAST

LUNCH

DINNER

SNACK 1

SNACK 2

TREATS

WATER

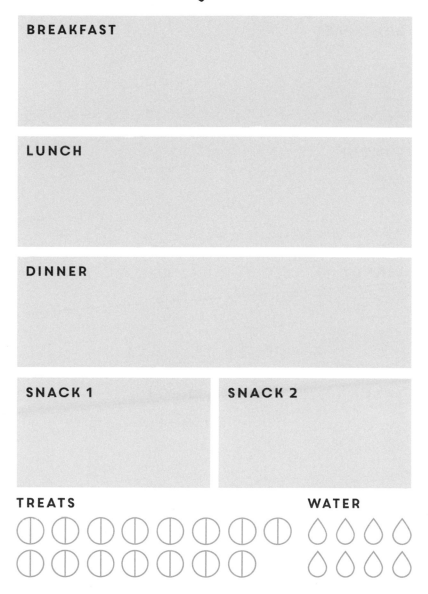

Day Four

BREAKFAST

LUNCH

DINNER

SNACK 1

SNACK 2

TREATS

WATER

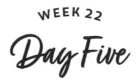

Day Five

BREAKFAST

LUNCH

DINNER

SNACK 1

SNACK 2

TREATS

WATER

Day Six

BREAKFAST

LUNCH

DINNER

SNACK 1

SNACK 2

TREATS

WATER

Day Seven

BREAKFAST

LUNCH

DINNER

SNACK 1

SNACK 2

TREATS

WATER

FOR COLOUR IMAGES OF THESE RECIPES, PLEASE VISIT PINCHOFNOM.COM /PLANNER

CHICKEN FOO YUNG

🕐 **10 MINS** | 🍲 **15 MINS** | 🔥 **287 KCAL** PER SERVING

The beauty of a good Foo Yung (Chinese omelette) recipe is that you can use whatever vegetables you have lying around. We've used classic Foo Yung vegetables in this recipe, but don't worry about swapping and changing them for whatever you have that needs using up.

Everyday Light

use GF soy sauce and stock cubes

GF

SERVES 4

low-calorie cooking spray
300g chicken breast (skin and visible fat removed), thinly sliced
3 tbsp light soy sauce
8 large eggs
sea salt and freshly ground black pepper
½ onion, sliced
½ red pepper, deseeded and sliced
150g beansprouts
3 spring onions, trimmed and thinly sliced
50g cooked peas

Spray a large frying pan or wok with low-calorie cooking spray, place over a high heat, add the chicken and stir-fry until almost cooked. Add 2 tablespoons of the soy sauce and continue stir-frying until it has almost evaporated. Transfer the cooked chicken to a bowl and set aside.

Crack the eggs into a bowl, beat lightly and season well with salt and pepper.

Return the frying pan or wok to the heat and spray it again with low-calorie cooking spray. Add the sliced onion and pepper and stir-fry for 3–4 minutes, then add the beansprouts and spring onions and stir-fry for another minute or two. Add the peas, chicken and remaining tablespoon of soy sauce. Mix, then add the beaten eggs and cook, stirring, until the egg has set – it should look like something between an omelette and scrambled eggs.

Remove from the heat and serve.

BEETROOT FALAFEL

🕐 **10 MINS** | 🍲 **25 MINS** | 💧 **238 KCAL** PER SERVING

Falafel are Middle Eastern bites of deliciousness! These are flavoured with an uncommon combination of feta and beetroot, but once you've tasted them, you'll wonder why everything in the world isn't made from these two ingredients! Filling and low in calories, these falafel will go down a storm.

Everyday Light

**MAKES 16 FALAFEL
(4 PER PORTION)**

low-calorie cooking spray
1 x 400g tin chickpeas,
   drained and rinsed
200g cooked beetroot
1 small onion, finely chopped
130g reduced-fat feta cheese,
   crumbled
1 tsp ground cumin
24 fresh mint leaves, chopped
salt and freshly ground black
   pepper

Preheat the oven to 200°C (fan 180°/gas mark 6) and spray a baking tray with low-calorie cooking spray.

Crush the chickpeas in a large mixing bowl with a fork.

Dry the beetroot, grate it into a bowl, then squeeze out any excess juice.

Spray a frying pan with low-calorie cooking spray, place over a medium heat and sauté the onion for 4–5 minutes, until soft and starting to brown.

Add the onion and grated beetroot to the crushed chickpeas, then add the feta, cumin and mint. Season well with salt and pepper and mix together.

Form the mixture into sixteen evenly sized balls and place them on the baking tray. Spray the falafel with low-calorie cooking spray and cook in the oven for 25 minutes.

Remove from the oven and serve warm. You can also allow to cool and freeze in an airtight container.

Week Twenty-Three

CHANGE +/-

CURRENT WEIGHT

THIS WEEK I WOULD LIKE TO ACHIEVE

LAST WEEK, THESE THINGS WENT WELL...

REMINDERS FOR THIS WEEK

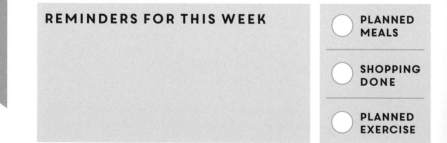

◯ PLANNED MEALS

◯ SHOPPING DONE

◯ PLANNED EXERCISE

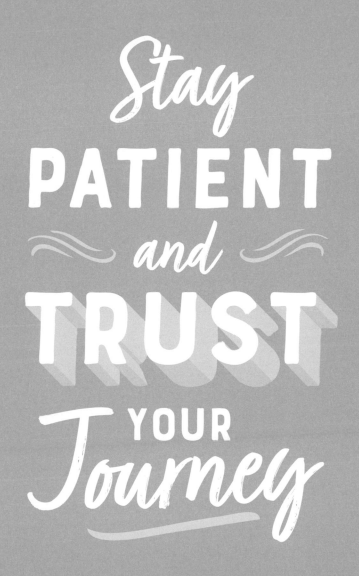

Day One

BREAKFAST

LUNCH

DINNER

SNACK 1

SNACK 2

TREATS

WATER

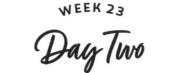

BREAKFAST

LUNCH

DINNER

SNACK 1

SNACK 2

TREATS

WATER

ROASTED TOMATO, FETA *and* SPINACH QUICHE

🕐 **10 MINS** | 🍲 **40 MINS** PLUS COOLING | 💧 **234 KCAL** PER SERVING

We've made a few crustless quiches in our time, but we have to say that this combination of ingredients is by far our favourite. Rich with feta and crammed full of filling spinach and juicy tomatoes, it's a simple recipe that will make a quick lunchtime meal a breeze!

Everyday Light

SERVES 4

low-calorie cooking spray
250g cherry tomatoes
½ tsp dried basil
200g spinach leaves
130g reduced-fat feta cheese
8 medium eggs
2 tbsp quark
sea salt and freshly ground
  black pepper

FOR COLOUR IMAGES OF THESE RECIPES, PLEASE VISIT PINCHOFNOM.COM /PLANNER

Preheat the oven to 200°C (fan 180°/gas mark 6). Place the tomatoes on a baking tray, spray with low-calorie cooking spray, sprinkle over the basil, and roast in the oven for 10 minutes.

Remove the tomatoes from the oven and turn down the oven to 190°C (fan 170°/gas mark 5).

Spray a frying pan with low-calorie cooking spray and place over a low heat. Add the spinach and stir until it wilts and releases its water, then tip it into a sieve and squeeze out as much excess water as possible.

Spray a 20cm (8in) quiche or flan dish with low-calorie cooking spray, place the spinach and roasted tomatoes in the dish then crumble over the feta.

Crack the eggs into a bowl, whisk in the quark and season well with salt and pepper. Pour the egg mixture into the quiche or flan dish, covering the feta, spinach and tomatoes, and transfer to the oven. Bake for 25–30 minutes, or until the quiche is set and golden on top. Remove from the oven and serve warm or cold.

QUICK-A-LILLI

🕐 **20 MINS** | 🍲 **3 MINS** | 🔥 **54 KCAL** PER SERVING

Originally a South Asian pickle, the English got hold of the idea in the 18th century, added some more seasoning and sauce, and created piccalilli. When we came up with this super-quick version and were considering what to call it, we had a eureka moment (it's a quick piccalilli … geddit?!).

Everyday Light

V **GF**

SERVES 6

200g cauliflower, cut into
   small florets
60g green beans, trimmed
   and cut into 1cm (½in) pieces
60g baby corn, cut into
   5mm (¼in) slices
180g courgettes, cut into
   1cm (½in) pieces
2 shallots, sliced
200ml cider vinegar
1 tsp ground turmeric
1 tsp English mustard powder
1 tsp garlic granules
1 tbsp granulated sweetener
¼–½ tsp xanthan gum
sea salt and freshly ground
   black pepper

Bring a large saucepan of salted water to the boil, then add the cauliflower florets. Bring back to the boil, add the green beans and corn, and cook for 1 minute, then add the courgettes and the shallots and cook for a further 30 seconds. Drain all the vegetables.

Put the vinegar, turmeric, mustard powder, garlic and sweetener in a small saucepan and heat gently until the sweetener has dissolved. Remove from the heat and whisk in the xanthan gum a little at a time until the liquid thickens just enough to coat the vegetables (whisk it well or it may go lumpy).

Mix the vegetables and the sauce together and add a little salt and pepper to taste.

It will keep well in the fridge in an airtight container for up to 3–4 days. Serve as an accompaniment to salads or cold meats.

Day Three

BREAKFAST

LUNCH

DINNER

SNACK 1

SNACK 2

TREATS

WATER

Day Four

BREAKFAST

LUNCH

DINNER

SNACK 1

SNACK 2

TREATS

WATER

Day Five

BREAKFAST

LUNCH

DINNER

SNACK 1

SNACK 2

TREATS

WATER

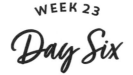

WEEK 23

Day Six

BREAKFAST

LUNCH

DINNER

SNACK 1

SNACK 2

TREATS

WATER

Day Seven

BREAKFAST

LUNCH

DINNER

SNACK 1

SNACK 2

TREATS

WATER

PANNA COTTA

⏱ **5 MINS** | 🍲 **5 MINS** PLUS CHILLING TIME | 💧 **123 KCAL** PER SERVING

Such a light dessert served with fruit; this quick sweet fix sent our taste testers wild. Try it and you'll understand why! It is absolutely ingenious. By using granulated sweetener and semi-skimmed milk, set with gelatine, you won't believe that this is easy on calories. But it really is!

———— *Special Occasion* ————

GF

SERVES 4

500ml semi-skimmed milk
3 tbsp granulated sweetener
1 vanilla pod
3 gelatine leaves
frozen berries, defrosted
    – raspberries are delish
icing sugar, for dusting
    (optional)

FOR A COLOUR IMAGE OF THIS RECIPE, PLEASE VISIT PINCHOFNOM.COM /PLANNER

Put the milk and sweetener in a small saucepan. Split the vanilla pod lengthways, scrape out the seeds and add them, and the split pod, to the milk. Heat gently to simmering point, stirring frequently, ensuring the milk doesn't catch and burn on the bottom of the pan.

While the milk is warming up, place the gelatine leaves in a bowl of cold water, ensuring the leaves are completely covered.

As soon as the milk reaches a simmer, remove the vanilla pod and take the pan off the heat. The gelatine leaves should now be soft. Squeeze them to remove any excess water and add them to the milk, mixing until they have dissolved.

Pour the mixture into four 12cm (4½ in) panna cotta or dariole moulds. Leave to cool, then place in the fridge for at least 2 hours (preferably overnight).

Run the tip of a knife carefully around the edge of each panna cotta and tip them out into dishes or plates. You might need to dip the mould briefly into some very hot water to encourage the panna cotta to come out. Top with your choice of berries and a dusting of icing sugar if desired.

Week Twenty-Four

CHANGE +/-

CURRENT WEIGHT

THIS WEEK I WOULD LIKE TO ACHIEVE

LAST WEEK, THESE THINGS WENT WELL...

REMINDERS FOR THIS WEEK

◯ **PLANNED MEALS**

◯ **SHOPPING DONE**

◯ **PLANNED EXERCISE**

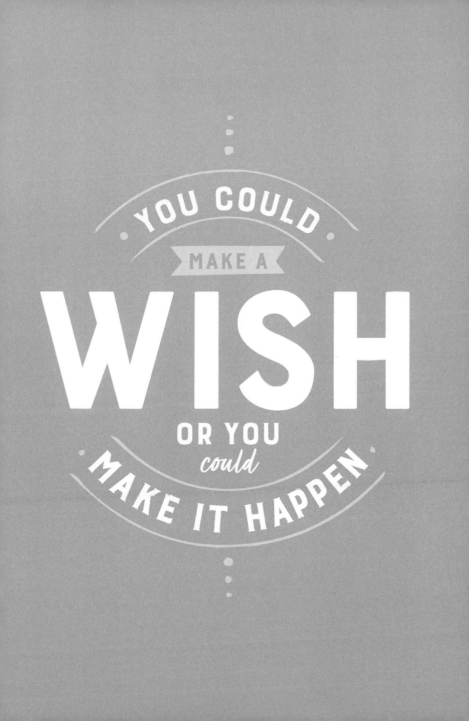

Day One

BREAKFAST

LUNCH

DINNER

SNACK 1

SNACK 2

TREATS

WATER

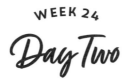

Day Two

BREAKFAST

LUNCH

DINNER

SNACK 1

SNACK 2

TREATS

WATER

Day Three

BREAKFAST

LUNCH

DINNER

SNACK 1

SNACK 2

TREATS

WATER

Day Four

BREAKFAST

LUNCH

DINNER

SNACK 1

SNACK 2

TREATS

WATER

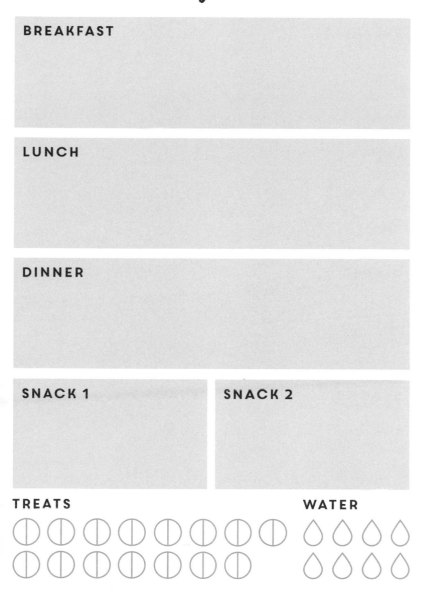

Day Five

BREAKFAST

LUNCH

DINNER

SNACK 1

SNACK 2

TREATS

WATER

Day Six

BREAKFAST

LUNCH

DINNER

SNACK 1

SNACK 2

TREATS

WATER

Day Seven

BREAKFAST

LUNCH

DINNER

SNACK 1

SNACK 2

TREATS

○ ○ ○ ○ ○ ○ ○ ○
○ ○ ○ ○ ○ ○ ○

WATER

◇ ◇ ◇ ◇
◇ ◇ ◇ ◇

CRISPY SEAWEED

FOR A COLOUR IMAGE OF THIS RECIPE, PLEASE VISIT PINCHOFNOM.COM /PLANNER

🕐 **2 MINS** | 🍲 **12 MINS** | 💧 **21 KCAL** PER SERVING

It's all a lie! The stuff you get from your local Chinese takeaway isn't really seaweed. Of course, you know that already. But that's why it's so easy to recreate. You don't need to don waders and head to the coast any time soon; a simple bag of cabbage will suffice! Add some decent seasoning and this will be a quick side dish you'll never need to order from the takeaway again.

Everyday Light

V **GF**

SERVES 4

low-calorie cooking spray
200g curly kale, stalks removed
1 tsp sea salt
1 tsp granulated sweetener
½ tsp garlic granules
½ tsp Chinese 5-spice

Preheat the oven to 220°C (fan 200°/gas mark 7) and spray a baking tray with low-calorie cooking spray.

Spread the kale out onto the baking tray and liberally spray it with low-calorie cooking spray. Sprinkle over the salt, sweetener, garlic and Chinese 5-spice, place the tray in the middle of the oven and bake for 4–5 minutes. Keep a close eye on it as you don't want it to burn!

Give the kale a mix, spread it out again, spray with more low-calorie cooking spray, return to the oven and bake for another 5–7 minutes, again watching to make sure it doesn't burn. When it is done it should be crispy around the edges but still look green.

Remove the tray from the oven and cut or break up the kale into smaller pieces. Now it's ready to serve.

Tip

TO GIVE THE KALE A LITTLE KICK, SPRINKLE WITH ½ TEASPOON DRIED CHILLI FLAKES BEFORE YOU PUT IT IN THE OVEN.

Week Twenty-Five

CHANGE +/-

CURRENT WEIGHT

THIS WEEK I WOULD LIKE TO ACHIEVE

LAST WEEK, THESE THINGS WENT WELL...

REMINDERS FOR THIS WEEK

- ◯ PLANNED MEALS
- ◯ SHOPPING DONE
- ◯ PLANNED EXERCISE

Day One

BREAKFAST

LUNCH

DINNER

SNACK 1

SNACK 2

TREATS

WATER

Day Two

BREAKFAST

LUNCH

DINNER

SNACK 1

SNACK 2

TREATS

WATER

Day Three

BREAKFAST

LUNCH

DINNER

SNACK 1

SNACK 2

TREATS

WATER

Day Four

BREAKFAST

LUNCH

DINNER

SNACK 1

SNACK 2

TREATS

WATER

Day Five

BREAKFAST

LUNCH

DINNER

SNACK 1

SNACK 2

TREATS

WATER

Day Six

BREAKFAST

LUNCH

DINNER

SNACK 1

SNACK 2

TREATS

WATER

Day Seven

BREAKFAST

LUNCH

DINNER

SNACK 1

SNACK 2

TREATS

WATER

New York
CHEESECAKE

🕐 **10 MINS** | 🍲 **45 MINS** PLUS COOLING | 💧 **212 KCAL** PER SERVING

A regular cheesecake usually consists of half fat, half sugar, so you may be surprised to see a cheesecake in this book! However, using quark is an amazing way to mimic that same creamy cheesecake consistency and taste without all the saturated fat – perfect! Using sweetener and vanilla extract in place of sugar, this amazing dessert keeps the calorie count right down as the taste goes up. Delicious!

—— *Special Occasion* ——

F

SERVES 8

6 reduced-fat digestive
  biscuits
25g reduced-fat spread
low-calorie cooking spray
175g reduced-fat soft cheese
500g quark
1 tsp vanilla extract or vanilla
  bean paste
4 large eggs
3 tbsp granulated sweetener
½ tsp xanthan gum

Preheat the oven to 160°C (fan 140°/gas mark 3).

Blitz the digestive biscuits in a food processor to form crumbs (or place them in a bag and crush them with a rolling pin). Tip the crumbs into the bottom of a 20cm (8in) loose-bottomed cake tin.

Melt the reduced-fat spread and pour it over the biscuit crumbs, mixing to ensure they're all coated. Press the crumbs down evenly to form the base of the cheesecake. Spray the biscuit base with low-calorie cooking spray and bake in the oven for 10 minutes.

Meanwhile, put all the remaining ingredients in a large mixing bowl and whisk together until smooth.

Remove the base from the oven, pour the cheesecake mix into the tin and put it back in the oven for 35 minutes, until the cheesecake is just set and starting to colour.

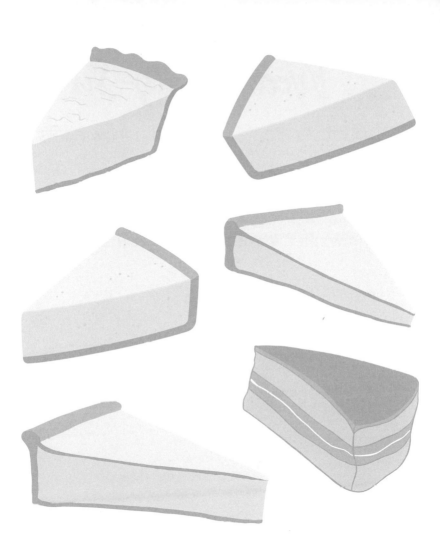

FOR A COLOUR IMAGE OF THIS RECIPE, PLEASE VISIT PINCHOFNOM.COM /PLANNER

Remove the cheesecake from the oven, leave it to cool in the tin, then refrigerate, preferably overnight.

Remove the chilled cheesecake from the tin and cut into slices to serve. You can also freeze the whole cheesecake in an airtight container.

Week Twenty-Six

CHANGE +/-

CURRENT WEIGHT

THIS WEEK I WOULD LIKE TO ACHIEVE

LAST WEEK, THESE THINGS WENT WELL...

REMINDERS FOR THIS WEEK

○ **PLANNED MEALS**

○ **SHOPPING DONE**

○ **PLANNED EXERCISE**

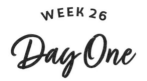

Day One

BREAKFAST

LUNCH

DINNER

SNACK 1

SNACK 2

TREATS

WATER

Day Two

BREAKFAST

LUNCH

DINNER

SNACK 1

SNACK 2

TREATS

WATER

Day Three

BREAKFAST

LUNCH

DINNER

SNACK 1

SNACK 2

TREATS

WATER

Day Four

BREAKFAST

LUNCH

DINNER

SNACK 1

SNACK 2

TREATS

WATER

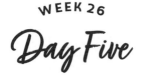

Day Five

BREAKFAST

LUNCH

DINNER

SNACK 1

SNACK 2

TREATS

WATER

Day Six

BREAKFAST

LUNCH

DINNER

SNACK 1

SNACK 2

TREATS

WATER

Day Seven

BREAKFAST

LUNCH

DINNER

SNACK 1

SNACK 2

TREATS

WATER

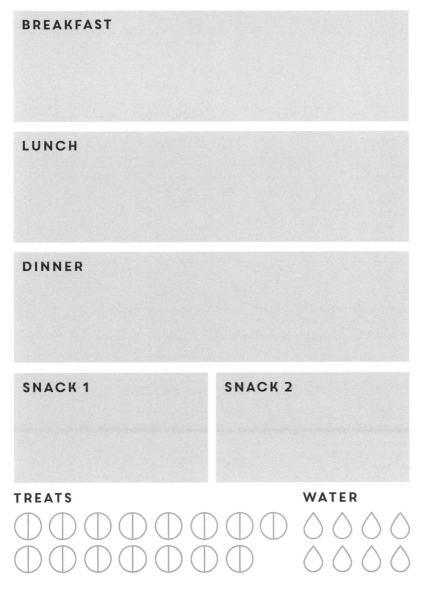

RECIPE INDEX

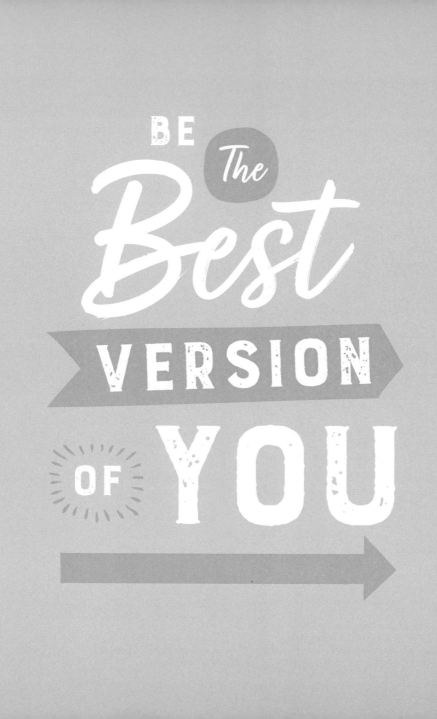

Notes

Notes

Thank
YOU

We want to say a huge thank you firstly, to all of our followers on social media and all those who make our recipes. Without you, this planner and everything else we do just wouldn't be possible.

Thank you to our publisher Carole, Martha, Bríd, Jodie and the rest of the team at Bluebird – you've been such an amazing part of the Pinch of Nom journey so far …!

Thanks to everyone at Nic & Lou, especially to Emma. You always take what is in our heads and make it look 1000 times better.

Special thanks go to Emma, Lisa and Meadows – thanks for all your hard work and your inspiration. Additional thanks go to Janie, Vince and Sydney – thank you for making Nom work and for keeping everything ticking over. We're so proud to work with you lot.

Our thanks also to our amazing taste testing group for all your help in sending feedback and suggestions for these recipes. We have really appreciated the time you gave to support this project.

Our agent Clare for believing in us from day one.

Thanks to Helen, Steve, Jen, Nick, Isla and Millie.

With thanks as ever to Paul – None of this would never have been possible without your and Cath's support. This, alongside everything we do, will always be for Cath.

No acknowledgement would be complete without a mention for our various furry babies – Brandi, Ginger Cat and Freda.

Your
ONLY
limit
IS YOU